LIPPINCOTT'S
POCKET
HISTOLOGY

LIPPINCOTT'S

POCKET
HISTOLOGY

Lisa M. J. Lee, PhD
Assistant Professor
University of Colorado School of Medicine
Department of Cell and Developmental Biology
Aurora, Colorado

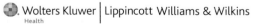

. Wolters Kluwer | Lippincott Williams & Wilkins
Health

Philadelphia · Baltimore · New York · London
Buenos Aires · Hong Kong · Sydney · Tokyo

Acquisitions Editor: Crystal Taylor
Product Manager: Lauren Pecarich
Marketing Manager: Joy Fisher Williams
Designer: Stephen Druding
Compositor: Aptara, Inc.

351 West Camden Street   Two Commerce Square
Baltimore, MD 21201   2001 Market Street
                                Philadelphia, PA 19103

Printed in China

9 8 7 6 5 4 3 2 1

Library of Congress Cataloging-in-Publication Data
Lee, Lisa M. J.
  Lippincott's pocket histology / Lisa M.J. Lee.
    p. ; cm.
  Pocket histology
  Includes index.
  ISBN 978-1-4511-7613-1
  I. Title. II. Title: Pocket histology.
  [DNLM: 1. Histology–Handbooks. QS 529]
  QM531
  611–dc23

                            2013009449

DISCLAIMER

I dedicate this book to my parents, whose unconditional love and sacrifice can never be fully repaid.

Health professions' curricula around the world are continually evolving: New discoveries, techniques, applications, and content areas compete for increasingly limited time with basic science topics. It is in this context that the foundations established in the basic sciences become increasingly important and relevant for absorbing and applying our ever-expanding knowledge of the human body. As a result of the progressively more crowded curricular landscape, students and instructors are finding new ways to maximize precious contact, preparation, and study time through more efficient, high-yield presentation and study methods.

Pocket Histology, as part of Lippincott's Pocket Series for the anatomical sciences, is designed to serve the time-crunched student. The presentation of histology in a table format featuring labeled images efficiently streamlines study and exam preparation for the highly visual and content-rich subject. This pocket-size, quick-reference book of histology pearls is portable, practical, and necessary; even at this small size, nothing is omitted and a large number of clinically significant facts, mnemonics, and easy-to-learn concepts are used to complement the tables and inform the reader.

I am confident that *Pocket Histology*, along with other books in the anatomical science Pocket Series, will greatly benefit all students attempting to learn clinically relevant foundational concepts in a variety of settings, including all graduate and professional health science programs.

ACKNOWLEDGMENTS

I would like to thank the student and faculty reviewers for their input into this book, which helped create a highly efficient learning and teaching tool. I would also like to thank Dr. Douglas Gould, who encouraged me to put my thoughts for *Pocket Histology* into reality and for his invaluable suggestions to producing this high-yield resource for students.

CONTENTS

Basic Principles of Histology | 1

INTRODUCTION

Histology (microanatomy) is the study of the human body at a tissue or sometimes at a cellular level. As disease processes occur at the molecular/cellular levels, manifestations of the disease processes are readily and economically observed at the tissue level using a microscope. To examine tissues under a microscope, several steps to acquire, fix, and stain the samples are necessary. In each of the preparatory steps, a variety of artifacts may be introduced to the tissue samples. A variety of staining agents and methods are available as are types of microscopes to help observe necessary cellular and histologic features.

BASIC PRINCIPLES

TECHNIQUES IN HISTOLOGY	
Methods	**Purpose**
Tissue preparation	
1. Tissue acquisition: Biopsy, surgical resection	1. Sampling tissue to examine microscopically
2. Fixation: Placing tissue samples in a fixative	2. Stopping tissue degradation, killing microorganisms
3. Processing: Series of chemical and heat treatment	3. Removing water from tissue, infiltrating the tissue with hardening agent
4. Embedding: Placing tissue into a hardening agent (paraffin) in a tissue block	4. Placing the tissue into rigid mold
5. Sectioning	5. Slicing the tissue into thin sections (7–12 μm)
6. Staining	6. Staining otherwise transparent tissues with different types of dyes or chemicals to observe cellular details

(continued)

TECHNIQUES IN HISTOLOGY (continued)

Methods	Purpose

Staining methods

1. Hematoxylin and eosin (H&E): Most common staining method using two dyes

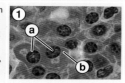

   a. Hematoxylin: Basic, positively charged dye

   b. Eosin: Acidic, negatively charged dye

2. Histochemistry: Staining chemicals bind or react with certain cellular structures

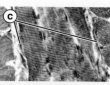

   c. Masson trichrome: Stains collagen and mucus blue, cytoplasm pink

   d. Periodic acid–Schiff (PAS): Polysaccharide such as glycogen turns dark red color.

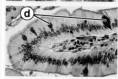

3. Immunohisto-chemistry: Applies specific antibody targeted at an antigen of interest and secondary antibody tagged with chemical agent that generates brown color

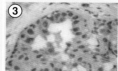

1. Staining basic or acidic structures of the tissue

   a. Purple to blue dye: Attracted to acidic, negatively charged cellular structures such as DNA and RNA in nuclei and on ribosomes in cytoplasm

   b. Pink to red dye: Attracted to basic, positively charged cellular structures (many proteins) in cytoplasm

2. Chemical reaction between the staining agent and tissue structures generates color.

   c. Identifies connective tissue content, organization, and makeup

   d. Identifies areas of high polysaccharide concentration such as basement membrane and goblet cells

3. Identifying cells or tissues that express the protein of interest

Methods		Purpose
Staining methods		
4. Immunofluorescence: Similar to immunohistochemistry in application of specific antibody, but the secondary antibody is tagged with fluorescent agent, can tag more than one specific protein with different color	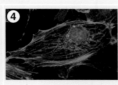	4. Identifying cells or tissues that express the protein of interest, may be able to tag more than one specific protein with different-colored fluorescence

Additional Concepts

- **Eosinophilia (acidophilia):** Tendency for cell or tissue structures to stain well with eosin, the acidic dye. Most cytoplasmic proteins are eosinophilic (acidophilic); they stain particularly well with eosin.
- **Basophilia:** Tendency for cell or tissue structures to stain well with hematoxylin, the basic dye. Nuclei, nucleoli, and cytoplasmic ribosomes are basophilic structures; they stain particularly well with hematoxylin.
- **Other naturally occurring pigments in cells**
  - **Melanin:** Black-brown pigments in certain types of cells such as keratinocytes of the skin
  - **Lipofuscin:** Yellow-brown pigment particles that accumulate in certain types of cells such as cardiomyocytes, neurons, and hepatocytes. Thought to be the residues of lysosomes
- **Artifacts:** Any artificial structures, defects, or observations that were introduced during preparatory steps and are not naturally present in vivo. Common artifacts observed in histologic tissue slides include dust particles, separation or folding of tissue slice, exaggeration of spaces between cells and tissues, and empty space effect in previously lipid-filled areas.

CYTOLOGY

Structure		Function	Location
Nucleus			
Oval to spherical, basophilic structure within most cells	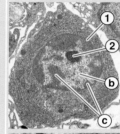	Storage of DNA and regulation of gene expression	Central to pericentral in most cells
1. Nuclear envelope: Two phospholipid bilayers		1. Forming a tightly controlled barrier between the nucleus and cytoplasm	1. Surrounding DNA content
a. Nuclear pore: Opening in nuclear envelope	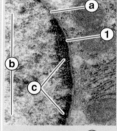	a. Regulating transport across nuclear envelope	a. Throughout nuclear envelope
2. Nucleolus: Small, round, basophilic structure		2. Ribosomal RNA (rRNA) assembly	2. Within nucleus of translationally active cells
3. Chromatin: DNA in organized spool form	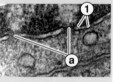	3. Organization of DNA	3. Within nucleus
b. Euchromatin: Unspooled chromatin, relatively pale staining areas of nucleus		b. Areas more accessible by transcription proteins	b. Transcriptionally active cells have more euchromatin than heterochromatin
c. Heterochromatin: Tightly spooled chromatin, darker staining areas of nucleus		c. Areas less accessible by transcription proteins	c. Transcriptionally inactive cells have more heterochromatin than euchromatin

Structure		Function	Location
Other major organelles			
1. Golgi: Stack of membrane-bound sacs		1. Posttranslational modification, sorting, packaging proteins	1. Perinuclear in most cells; well developed in secretory, translationally active cells
a. Cis-face: Flattened sacs		a. Receiving newly formed proteins	a. Closer to nucleus
b. Trans-face: Curved sacs		b. Sending out modified proteins to appropriate locations in the cell	b. Farther from nucleus
2. Mitochondria: Spherical to elongated oval structure with two membranes		2. Large amount of adenosine triphosphate (ATP) generation	2. Numerous in cells that generate and expand much energy
c. Outer membrane: Smooth outer layer		c. Forming an outer boundary, containing ATP transporters	c. Outer layer of mitochondria
d. Inner membrane with cristae, complex infoldings		d. Containing machineries for aerobic respiration and large amount of ATP generation	d. Inner layer of mitochondria

(continued)

CYTOLOGY (continued)

Structure		Function	Location
Other major organelles			
3. Rough endoplasmic reticulum (rER): Series of membrane-bound tubules and sacs with ribosomes on the outside	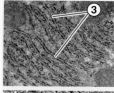	3. Protein synthesis	3. Abundant in translationally active, secretory cells
4. Smooth endoplasmic reticulum (sER): Series of membrane-bound tubules without ribosomes		4. Producing membrane materials, lipid metabolism	4. Abundant in cells involved in lipid metabolism
Cytoskeleton			
Collection of filamentous fibers in various orientations in a cell	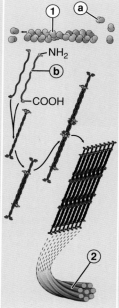	Providing structural support, mechanism for cellular movements, scaffolding and anchoring for organelles; participating in intracellular trafficking	Throughout cell cytoplasm
1. Actin filaments: Thin filaments 6–8 nm in diameter; lengths vary a. Actin monomer subunits		1. Locomotion of cells, cellular processes; forming structural core of microvilli	1. Abundant in muscles within contractile machinery, core of microvilli
2. Intermediate filaments: Rope-like filaments 8–10 nm in diameter		2. Supporting, providing general structural scaffolding to a cell	2. Throughout cytoplasm in most cells

Structure	Function	Location
Cytoskeleton		
Many different types are present but are expressed in a tissue-specific manner		
b. Eight tetramers of filamentous monomer protein		
3. Microtubules: Hollow tubular protein fibers 20–25 nm in diameter composed of tubulin proteins	3. Intracellular transportation, generation of cell motility	3. Throughout cytoplasm
a. Centriole: Cylinder of short nine microtubule triplets	a–b. Controlling microtubule formation	a–b. Close to nucleus
b. Centrosome: Two centrioles at right angle to each other		
c. Axoneme: Cylinder of nine microtubule doublets with two single microtubules in the center	c. Movement of cilia, flagella	c. Core of cilia and flagella

Additional Concepts

- **Tissue-specific intermediate filaments:** There are several different types of intermediate filaments and they are expressed in a tissue-specific manner (i.e., keratin intermediate filaments are only expressed in epithelial-derived cells and vimentin intermediate filaments are only expressed in mesenchymal-derived cells). Such specificity is useful when identifying the tissue origin of metastatic or dedifferentiated tumors.
- **Cytologic features indicating cellular activity:** Large nucleus; general euchromasia; distinct, large nucleolus (sometimes more than one); well-developed Golgi; and basophilic cytoplasm indicating abundant RNA associated with ribosomes all hint at rich transcriptional and translational activity of the cell. On the other hand, small and mostly heterochromatic nucleus, indistinct nucleolus, and scant cytoplasm indicate cellular inactivity.

MICROSCOPY		
Type	**Function**	
Light	1. Standard microscopy utilizing natural light to observe tissues stained with H&E, other histochemistry and immunohistochemistry a. Phase contrast microscopy: Utilizes slight refractory differences between cellular parts to observe unstained tissues and live cells	
Fluorescence	2. Used to observe fluorescently dyed tissues (immunofluorescence), utilizing UV rays or lasers to excite the fluorescence-tagged epitopes	
Confocal	3. Capable of focusing on a single plane within a tissue, reducing the noise created by other layers within the tissue	

Type	Function
Electron	4. Utilizes electrons rather than photons to observe cellular structures at much higher resolution a. Scanning electron microscopy allows observation of surface features b. Transmission electron microscopy allows observation of cellular structures in 2-dimension

Epithelial Tissue | 2

INTRODUCTION

Epithelial tissue is one of the four basic tissue types composed of diverse morphologic and functional subtypes that cover body surfaces, line body cavities, and form a variety of glands. The unique feature of the epithelial tissues is its highly cellular composition with little extracellular matrix (ECM), which makes cell–cell adhesion and communication very important for the integrity and function of the epithelium. Epithelial tissues rest on top of the basement membrane, which separates epithelia from underlying connective tissues. Because epithelia are avascular, they are heavily dependent on diffusion of nutrients from the underlying connective tissue and have a limit on its thickness. The organization and types of cells in epithelial tissue determine its classification and function (FIGURE 2-1), which varies from protection to absorption and secretion.

EPITHELIAL TISSUE

EPITHELIAL INTEGRITY		
Structure	Function	Location
Cell–cell junctions		
1. Zonula occludens (occluding, tight, impermeable junction): Cell membranes of adjacent cells are in contact with each other, forming a web-like seal	1. Sealing epithelial cells together, preventing paracellular diffusion of materials, maintaining cell polarity	1. Apical-most level of the lateral cell membrane

(continued)

EPITHELIAL INTEGRITY (continued)

Structure		Function	Location
Cell–cell junctions			

2. Zonula adherens (adhesion junctions): Band-like adhesion sites, close adjacent cell membranes, fuzzy plaques on cytoplasmic membrane made of actin filaments

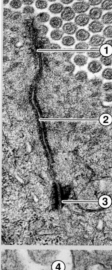

2. Reinforcing cell–cell adhesion, resisting separation between cells

2. Immediately below zonula occludens on lateral cell membrane

3. Desmosomes (macula adherens): Space between adjacent cells with electron-dense line, dense plaque of intermediate filaments on cytoplasmic membrane

3. Anchoring adjacent cells together, reinforcing cell–cell adhesion, resisting separation

3. Scattered throughout lateral membrane below zonula adherens

4. Gap junctions (communicating junctions): Adjacent cell membranes are in close proximity

4. Allowing direct passage of signaling molecules between cells

4. Scattered throughout lateral membrane below zonula adherens

Structure		Function	Location
Cell-connective tissue junctions			
5. Hemidesmo-somes: Intracellular plaque similar to desmosomes with intermediate filaments		5. Anchoring epithelia to basement membrane and connective tissue, resisting abrasion and force to prevent separation between epithelium and connective tissue	5. Basal cell surface

Clinical Significance

- **Bullous pemphigoid:** Chronic blistering skin disease most commonly resulting from autoantibodies that bind the skin's basement membrane, initiating inflammatory reaction that breaks down hemidesmosomal proteins. Patients present with numerous, large, painful blisters as the result of epidermal separation from the underlying connective tissue.
- **Pemphigus:** Chronic blistering skin disease similar to bullous pemphigoid, but the autoantibodies bind the keratinocyte desmosomes, resulting in a loss of cell–cell adhesions and blisters within the epidermis as the epithelial cells separate from each other. Hemidesmosomes are intact and maintains contact with the basement membrane.

EPITHELIAL CLASSIFICATION			
Criteria/ Structure		Function	Location
Number of cell layers			
1. Simple: Single cell layer		1. Lining body cavities or glands, absorption, secretion	1. Areas that require quick transport of materials, large amount of absorption and secretion

(continued)

EPITHELIAL CLASSIFICATION (continued)

Criteria/ Structure		Function	Location
Number of cell layers			
2. Stratified: More than one layer of cells		2. Lining, protecting areas of the body that need more strength and resistance	2. Areas that require protection and strength
3. Pseudostratified: Cells appear stratified, but every cell contacts basement membrane		3. Lining, absorption, secretion, creating current across epithelium	3. Areas that require movement of secretion or fluids, absorption and secretion
Shape of the apical cells			
1. Squamous: Flat cells with thin and wide cytoplasm and nuclei	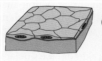	1. Fast transport of molecules across cytoplasm, or protection in many layers	1. Areas that require rapid exchange of molecules or protection in many layers
2. Cuboidal: Cube-shaped cells with central, spherical nuclei		2. Relatively fast absorption and secretion	2. Some exocrine and endocrine glands, ducts
3. Columnar: Rectangular, tall cells with central to basal, oval nuclei		3. Large amount of absorption and secretion	3. Lining of the intestine and respiratory tract

Criteria/ Structure		Function	Location
Transitional epithelium			
Number of layers and shape of the cells change based on distention of the organ		Allowing distension and recoil of an organ	Urinary bladder, ureter, calyces, urethra
Apical specialization			
1. Keratinization: Layer of flattened, dead cells		1. Forming protective layer against force, friction, desiccation	1. Areas exposed to repeated and prolonged exposure to force, friction, and air
2. Microvilli: Short, numerous cellular projections		2. Increasing surface area of the luminal border	2. Areas that require large amount of absorption and secretion
3. Cilia: Specialized cellular projections with motile mechanisms		3. Generating movements to create current	3. Areas that require movement of fluids over the epithelium
4. Stereocilia: Long, immotile cellular projections		4. Increasing surface area for absorption, serving as mechanoreceptors	4. Epididymis, special sensory epithelium

Epithelial Classification Formula

Surface + Number of + Apical cell = _____ epithelium
specialization   cell layers   morphology

↓   ↓   ↓

Stratified { • Keratinized   • Simple   • Squamous
squamous { • Nonkeratinized   • Stratified   • Cuboidal
only   • Pseudostratified • Columnar

Columnar { • Ciliated   • Transitional
only   { • Nonciliated

Figure 2-1. The organization and types of cells in epithelial tissue determine its classification and function.

TYPES OF EPITHELIA

Structure		Function	Location
Simple squamous epithelium			
1. Single layer of flattened cells	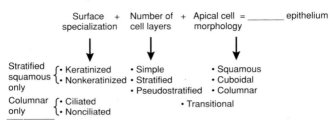	1. Rapid exchange of gas; small, lipid-soluble molecules; and fluid	1. Luminal lining of vessels, lung alveoli, body cavity serous lining
Simple cuboidal epithelium			
2. Single layer of cube-shaped cells	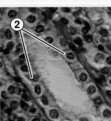	2. Relatively quick absorption, secretion	2. Kidney tubules, pancreatic acini, small ducts, thyroid follicles

Structure		Function	Location
Simple columnar epithelium			
3. Single layer of rectangular cells		3. Large amount of absorption, secretion, protection	3. Lining and glands of majority of gastrointestinal (GI) tracts
Ciliated simple columnar epithelium			
4. Single layer of rectangular cells with cilia on apical surface		4. Absorption, secretion, generation of current across the epithelium	4. Lining of fallopian tube
Ciliated pseudostratified columnar epithelium			
5. Single layer of ciliated columnar cells, other types of cells intermixed		5. Absorption, secretion, generation of current across the epithelium	5. Most of respiratory tract
Keratinized stratified squamous epithelium			
6. Thick layer of cells a. Cuboidal cells on basement membrane b. Flattened, eosinophilic, anucleate cells on apical surface		6. Protection from repeated, prolonged exposure to force and friction, preventing desiccation	6. Skin

(continued)

TYPES OF EPITHELIA (continued)

Structure	Function	Location
Nonkeratinized stratified squamous epithelium		
7. Thick layer of cells; cuboidal cells on basement membrane 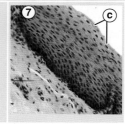 c. Flattened, but-nucleated cells on apical surface	7. Protection from repeated, prolonged exposure to force and friction	7. Oral cavity, esophagus, vagina, anal canal
Stratified cuboidal epithelium		
8. Two or more layers of cuboidal cells 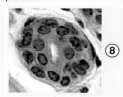	8. Maintaining the shape and patency of ducts	8. Interlobular and intralobular ducts
Stratified columnar epithelium		
9. Two or more layers of rectangular cells 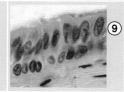	9. Maintaining the shape and patency of larger ducts	9. Terminal ducts
Transitional epithelium		
10. More than one layer of polygonal cells 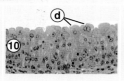 d. Dome cells: Rounded, sometimes binucleate cells protruding out into the lumen on apical surface	10. Reducing number of layers and flattening the cells as the organ distends, then recoiling back to normal shape	10. Lining of calyces, renal pelvis, ureter, urinary bladder, portions of urethra

Additional Concepts

- **Endothelium:** Simple squamous epithelium that lines the lumen of the vessels.
- **Mesothelium:** Simple squamous epithelium that lines the serous membrane of the body cavities.
- **Respiratory epithelium:** Ciliated pseudostratified columnar epithelium that lines most of the conducting portions of the respiratory system.
- **Turnover:** Epithelia have the highest turnover rate out of the four basic tissue types. The turnover rate varies depending on location and function; skin epithelium turns over every 30 days and colonic mucosal epithelium turns over every week. With the high turnover rate, susceptibility for acquiring mutations and developing neoplasm is also the highest out of the four tissue types.
- **Lining versus glandular epithelium:**
  - **Lining epithelia:** Cover the surface of the skin or body cavity that are in direct contact with the luminal space.
  - **Glandular epithelia:** Involved in production of secretions released into the lumen or nearby blood vessels. Glandular epithelia are not in direct contact with luminal space and are embedded in connective tissues, separated by the basement membrane.

GLANDS			
Structure		**Function**	**Location**
Exocrine glands			
Secrete into the lumen directly or via the duct			
1. Unicellular: Single goblet-shaped cell within lining epithelium		1. Mucous secretion	1. Scattered within lining epithelia of respiratory tract and GI tract

(continued)

GLANDS (continued)

Structure		Function	Location
Exocrine glands			
2. Simple tubular: Test-tube-shaped glands a. Secretory unit: Simple columnar epithelium		2. Mucous secretion	2. Small and large intestine
3. Simple branched tubular: More than one test-tube-shaped gland sharing a common duct or opening into lumen b. Secretory units: Simple columnar epithelium		3. Mostly mucous secretion	3. Stomach pylorus

4. Simple coiled tubular: Long, convoluted gland
  c. Secretory unit: Simple cuboidal to stratified cuboidal epithelium; larger, pale staining cells
  d. Duct: Stratified cuboidal epithelium; smaller, darker staining cells
		4. Sweat secretion	4. Skin sweat glands

Structure		Function	Location
Exocrine glands			
5. Simple acinar: Single spherical gland draining into a short duct		5. Mucous secretion	5. Glands of Litre near penile ure-thra
e. Secretory unit: Simple cuboi-dal to colum-nar epithelium			
6. Simple branched acinar: More than one spheri-cal gland draining into a common duct		6. Sebum secretion	6. Skin seba-ceous glands
f. Secretory unit: Stratified cuboidal epi-thelium, cells are large and vacuolated			
7. Compound tubu-lar: More than one tubular gland and more than one duct opening into lumen		7. Mucous secretion	7. Brunner glands of duodenum
g. Secretory unit: Simple columnar epithelium, pale-staining cells			
h. Ducts: Simple columnar epithelium, dark-staining cells			
8. Compound aci-nar: More than one spherical gland, more than one duct of vary-ing size		8. Watery protein-aceous secretion	8. Parotid glands, pan-creas, mam-mary glands

(continued)

GLANDS (continued)		
Structure	**Function**	**Location**
Exocrine glands		
i. Secretory units: Simple cuboidal to pyramidal, mostly serous secreting cells filled with secretory granules 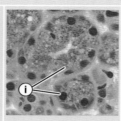		
j. Ducts: Simple cuboidal, simple columnar, stratified columnar		
9. Compound tubuloacinar: More than one tubular and spherical gland, more than one duct of varying size 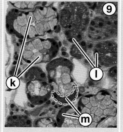	9. Mucous and serous secretion	9. Submandibular and sublingual salivary glands
k. Simple columnar secretory units		
l. Simple cuboidal secretory units		
m. Demilunes: Simple columnar tubular glands capped at the end by the hemispherical simple cuboidal acinar gland		
n. Ducts: Simple cuboidal, simple columnar, stratified columnar		

Structure	Function	Location
Endocrine glands		
Secrete into nearby capillary network, no ducts present	Signal distant target cells to respond to hormonal signals	
1. Unicellular: Single cells often within glandular epithelia, subnuclear secretory vesicles released into underlying connective tissue	1. Release of hormones affecting the epithelium they reside in	1. Scattered throughout GI tract
2. Cords: Plates of polygonal cells supported by reticular tissue and surrounded by abundant capillaries	2. Release of various hormones	2. Pituitary, parathyroid, and adrenal glands; islets of Langerhans
3. Follicles: Spherical secretory units lined by simple cuboidal endocrine cells, filled with gelatinous colloid	3. Storage of iodide, production and secretion of thyroid hormones	3. Thyroid gland

Additional Concepts

- **Exocrine versus endocrine glands:** Both derive from lining epithelial cells that proliferate and invaginate into underlying connective tissue. Whereas exocrine glands maintain their connection to the lining epithelium via ducts, endocrine glands lose the connection when the ducts degenerate. Exocrine glands release their products to the luminal space of an organ via ducts, whereas endocrine glands release their products within the body via nearby capillary networks.

HISTOLOGIC LOOK-A-LIKES

	Simple Columnar Epithelium	Pseudostratified Squamous Epithelium	Transitional Epithelium
Nuclei	Relatively even, single row of oval nuclei	Uneven, oval nuclei; difficult to discern a row or rows of nuclei, but pooled toward basal layer	Spherical nuclei scattered throughout the entire thickness of epithelium, uneven, no discernible rows
Apical layer	Relatively distinct, clean boundary	Ciliated	Dome-shaped cells protruding out to luminal space

Connective Tissue | 3

INTRODUCTION

Connective tissue is one of the four basic tissue types composed of diverse morphologic and functional subtypes found in a variety of locations ranging from dermis, mesenteries, and tendons to cartilage, bone, and blood. The common characteristic of connective tissue is its composition; relatively sparse cells embedded or suspended in an abundant extracellular matrix (ECM), which is a mixture of fibers, ground substance, and a varying amount of water. The ECM content and the types of cells in connective tissue determine its structure, function, and classification. Connective tissues in general provide structural, nutritional, immunologic, and communicational support to the surrounding tissues and/or organs.

CONNECTIVE TISSUE

CONNECTIVE TISSUE COMPONENTS			
Structure		**Function**	**Location**
Cells			
		Provide functions of the connective tissue	
1. Fibroblasts: Dendritic to fusiform cells with oval, euchromatic nuclei		1. Produce fibers	1. Throughout connective tissue, close to fibers

(continued)

CONNECTIVE TISSUE COMPONENTS (continued)

Structure		Function	Location
Cells			
2. Fibrocytes: Flat, fusiform cells with thin, heterochromatic nuclei	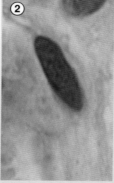	2. Maintain fibers	2. Throughout connective tissue, close to mature fibers
3. Adipocytes: Spherical cells with large lipid droplets and peripherally displaced, flattened nuclei	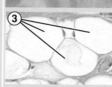	3. Store lipids, cushion and insulate nearby structures	3. Throughout connective tissue, abundant in adipose connective tissue
4. Mast cells: Large, ovoid cells with spherical nuclei and abundant dark-brown granules		4. Produce and secrete inflammatory mediators such as histamine	4. Throughout connective tissue, abundant in dermis and mucosal lamina propria

Structure		Function	Location
Cells			
5. Macrophages: Various sizes and shapes, often difficult to identify		5. Phagocytose pathogens and debris	5. Throughout connective tissue
6. Plasma cells: Oval cells with eccentric "clock face" nuclei, perinuclear clearing due to Golgi, basophilic cytoplasm		6. Produce antibodies	6. Throughout connective tissue, abundant in mucosal lamina propria
7. Eosinophils: Bilobed nuclei, eosinophilic granule-filled cytoplasm		7. Immune function: Mediators of allergic response and parasitic infection response	7. Throughout connective tissue, circulate in blood
8. Lymphocytes: Relatively small oval cells, clear cytoplasm, dense nuclei		8. Immune function: Major role in adaptive response	8. Throughout connective tissue, abundant at the site of chronic inflammation, circulate in blood

(continued)

CONNECTIVE TISSUE COMPONENTS (continued)

Structure	Function	Location

Cells

Structure	Function	Location
9. Neutrophils: Nuclei with three to four lobes, granular cytoplasm 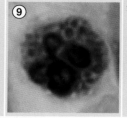	9. Immune function: Acute inflammatory response	9. Throughout connective tissue, abundant at the site of acute inflammation, circulate in blood

Fibers

Structure	Function	Location
1. Collagen fibers: Thick, eosinophilic, long, rope-like strands mostly composed of type I collagen 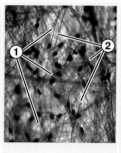	1. Provide flexibility, structural support, and strength to the tissue	1. Scattered throughout connective tissues; abundant in bones, tendons, ligaments
2. Elastic fibers: Thin, dark, long, branched, hair-like strands composed of elastin and fibrillin	2. Provide elasticity, give the tissue the ability to distend and recoil	2. Scattered throughout connective tissues; abundant in large arteries, dermis
3. Reticular fibers: Very thin, short, type III fibrillar strands. Not visible without special stain 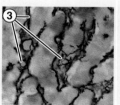	3. Provide a delicate meshwork and supporting scaffolding for cells and other fibers in a tissue	3. Scattered throughout connective tissues; abundant in lymph nodes, spleen, glands

Structure		Function	Location
Ground substance			
1. Viscous, gel-like substance with high water content; appears as clear, nonstaining areas. Major components: Proteoglycans, multiadhesive glycoproteins, glycosaminoglycans	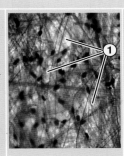	1. Contribute to mechanical and structural support, anchor fibers and cells in respective areas of the tissue, allow diffusion of nutrients and chemicals throughout the tissue	1. Throughout connective tissue; in between fibers and cells

CONNECTIVE TISSUE PROPER

Structure		Function	Location
Loose (areolar) connective tissue			
Relatively cellular connective tissue with all three types of loosely arranged fibers and abundant ground substance. Well vascularized		Support, cushion, and deliver vascular supply to the nearby epithelia. Immediately respond to epithelial injury or contact with antigens	Commonly under epithelia; throughout dermis, lamina propria, layers surrounding glands and ducts
1. Fibers: Sparse, irregularly arranged a. Collagen: Thick, long, eosinophilic, rope-like type I strands	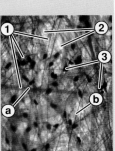	1. Provide structural support, elasticity, protection a. Provide strength and structural support	Fibers, ground substance, and cells are scattered throughout the tissue

(continued)

CONNECTIVE TISSUE PROPER (continued)

Structure	Function	Location

Loose (areolar) connective tissue

b. Elastic: Thin, dark, long, branched, hair-like strands composed of elastin and fibrillin

    b. Provide elasticity

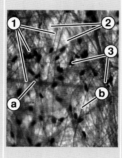

c. Reticular fibers: Very thin, short, type III fibrillar strands. Not visible without special stain

    c. Provide a meshwork of scaffolds for cells and fibers

2. Abundant ground substance: Nonstaining areas of the tissue

    2. Attract water into ECM, provide structural strength, allow diffusion of molecules, stabilize position of fibers and cells

3. Diverse cell types scattered throughout

    3. Provide a variety of functions of the connective tissue

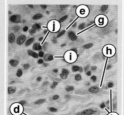

d. Fibroblasts: Dendritic to fusiform cells with oval, euchromatic nucleus

    d. Produce fibers

e. Fibrocytes: Flat, fusiform cells with thin, heterochromatic nucleus

    e. Maintain fibers

Structure	Function	Location
Loose (areolar) connective tissue		
f. Adipocytes: Spherical cells with large lipid droplets and peripherally displaced, flattened nucleus	f. Store lipids	
g. Mast cells: Large, ovoid cells with spherical nuclei and abundant dark-brown granules	g. Produce and secrete inflammatory mediators such as histamine	
h. Macrophages	h. Phagocytose pathogens and debris	
i. Plasma cells	i. Produce antibodies	
j. Eosinophils	j. Immune function: Mediators of allergic response and parasitic infection response	
k. Lymphocytes	k. Immune function: Major role in adaptive response	
l. Neutrophils	l. Immune function: Acute inflammatory response	

(continued)

CONNECTIVE TISSUE PROPER (continued)

Structure	Function	Location

Dense irregular connective tissue

Composed of densely packed mostly collagen fibers in diverse orientations with much less ground substance and sparse fibrocytes

1. Collagen fibers: Thick, eosinophilic, rope-like strands cut in various planes due to irregular arrangements

2. Fibrocytes: Thin, dark, condensed nuclei scattered sparsely throughout tissue

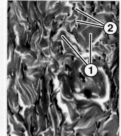
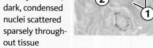

Provide structural support and strength to withstand force applied from multiple directions

1. Provide structural support, tensile strength

2. Produce and maintain fibers

Deeper layer of dermis (reticular dermis) and submucosa

Dense regular connective tissue

Composed of densely packed collagen fibers arranged in parallel bundles with sparse ground substance and fibrocytes wedged in between fibers

1. Collagen fibers: Thick, eosinophilic, rope-like strands in linear arrangements

2. Fibrocytes: Thin, dark, condensed nuclei scattered sparsely throughout tissue, parallel to fibers

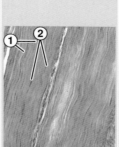

Provide structural support and strength to withstand force applied in one direction (the direction of the fiber orientation)

1. Provide structural support, tensile strength

2. Produce and maintain fibers

Tendons, ligaments, aponeuroses

SPECIALIZED CONNECTIVE TISSUE

Structure	Function	Location
Elastic connective tissue		
Composed of parallel layers of elastic fibers interspersed with fibrocytes, other fibers, and smooth muscle cells	Provide structural support while allowing certain level of distension and recoil	Large arteries, certain vertebral ligaments
1. Elastic fibers: Thin, wavy, branching, hair-like strands in parallel layers 2. Fibrocytes and smooth muscles	1. Provide elasticity and flexibility to allow stretching and recoil 2. Produce fibers and aid in recoil	
Reticular connective tissue		
Composed of a meshwork of predominantly reticular fibers, fair amount of ground substance, reticulocytes (reticular cells, fibroblasts), and parenchymal cells	Provide structural scaffold for relatively soft organs that functionally require a large capillary/lymph network or organs composed mostly of secretory cells	Liver, spleen, lymph nodes, pancreas, bone marrow, salivary glands, endocrine glands
1. Reticular fibers: Thin, short, fibrillar fibers that form a net-like meshwork 2. Reticulocytes: Dendritic to fusiform specialized fibroblasts	1. Provide structural scaffold for an organ 2. Produce and maintain reticular fibers	

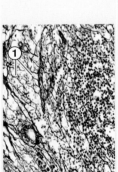

(continued)

SPECIALIZED CONNECTIVE TISSUE (continued)

Structure	Function	Location
Unilocular (white) adipose tissue		
Composed mostly of unilocular adipocytes: Large spherical cells with a large, single, lipid-filled globule taking up most of the cytoplasmic space with a perinuclear, flattened nucleus 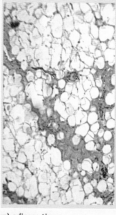	Lipid storage, insulation, and protection	Throughout the adult body, hypodermis, mesentery, omentum, and other visceral fat pads
Multilocular (brown) adipose tissue		
Composed mostly of multilocular adipocytes: Large spherical cells with abundant, small, lipid-filled vesicles in cytoplasm; central nuclei; abundant mitochondria 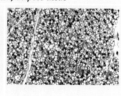	Heat generation	Throughout the body of the embryo and infants
Mesenchymal tissue		
Loosely arranged and delicate embryonic connective tissue composed of:	Form embryonic connective tissue from which other types of tissue may arise	Throughout developing embryo

Structure	Function	Location
Mesenchymal tissue		
1. Network of mesenchymal cells: Uniform dendritic to spindle-shaped cells	1. Produce ECM, may differentiate into different types of cells	
2. Large amount of ground substance: Pale-staining regions	2. Provide structural support	
3. Mostly reticular fibers	3. Provide structural scaffolding	
Blood: Covered in *Cardiovascular System*		

Additional Concepts

- **Vascularity:**
  - Loose connective tissues: Commonly found under avascular epithelial tissues; are highly vascular; serve as the main nutritional supply to the epithelia as well as a primary site of immune response in case of injury or infection
  - Dense regular connective tissues: Are not as vascular; hence, injuries to tendons or ligaments tend to heal slowly.
- **Mesenchyme:** The specialized connective tissue of the developing embryo and fetus. Common misconception is that mesenchyme derives from the mesoderm, but this is incorrect. Mesenchyme may derive from any of the three germ layers (ectoderm, mesoderm, and endoderm).
- **Interstitial fluid dynamics:** Since water is one of the major components of the ECM, fluid homeostasis in the connective tissue is extremely important. The balance is maintained by the hydrostatic pressure of the arterioles that initially forces the water out into the interstitium and the osmotic pressure of the terminal capillaries and venules that draws water back into the vessels. Excess interstitial fluid is drained by the lymphatic vessels and is returned to the circulatory system. Disruption of any aspect of this balance may result in edema and excess accumulation of fluid in the tissue.

Clinical Significance

- **Anaphylaxis:** An acute inflammatory reaction involving multiple organs as the result of mast cell and basophil degranulation in response to an allergen exposure. Resulting airway edema, bronchospasm, vasodilation, and increased vascular permeability may be fatal to the patient if not treated immediately. Emergency administration of epinephrine helps to maintain blood pressure and antagonize the inflammatory mediators.
- **Marfan syndrome:** Commonly caused by the abnormal fibrillin expression resulting in abnormal and insufficient elastic fiber formation. Patients tend to exhibit characteristic phenotypic features such as tall stature, caved-in chest, long fingers, and increased susceptibility to ectopia of the lens and aortic dissection.
- **Scurvy:** Vitamin C deficiency that results in impaired collagen formation, negatively affecting connective tissues and organs with high collagen content, thus weakening bones, skin, and oral mucosa

SUPPORTING CONNECTIVE TISSUE: CARTILAGE		
Structure	Function	Location
Hyaline cartilage		
Firm, solid, and rigid tissue with limited pliability	Provide structural support, rigidity, and protection to soft tissues in the vicinity. Provide low-friction joint surfaces and distribute force	Costal cartilages, articular surfaces, epiphyseal plates, nose
1. Chondrocytes: Ovoid cells with eccentric round nuclei located within: a. Lacunae: Small spaces fairly evenly spaced 	1. Produce and maintain cartilage ECM a. House chondrocytes	1. Throughout cartilage inside lacunae a. Throughout cartilage

Structure		Function	Location
Hyaline cartilage			
2. ECM: Composed mostly of type II collagen and glycosaminoglycans; appear homogenous, glassy		2. Attract water that provides resilience and allows diffusion of metabolites throughout avascular cartilage tissue	2. In between chondrocytes
3. Perichondrium: Dense connective tissue containing:		3. Surround, protect, and deliver nutrients to cartilage	3. Outside of the cartilage
b. Chondroblasts: Resemble fibrocytes		b. Differentiate into chondrocytes	b. Within perichondrium, usually in a layer closer to cartilage
c. Fibroblasts/ fibrocytes: Dendritic to spindle cells		c. Produce ECM of the perichondrium	c. Throughout perichondrium, usually in the outer layer
d. Blood vessels		d. Supply cartilage with nutrients and oxygen	d. Throughout perichondrium
Elastic cartilage			
Firm, solid tissue with flexibility and elasticity that contains:		Provide structural support and rigidity but also a range of flexibility and elasticity to change shape and return to the original form and position	Pinna of the external ear, external auditory meatus, auditory (eustachian) tube, epiglottis

(continued)

SUPPORTING CONNECTIVE TISSUE: CARTILAGE (continued)

Structure		Function	Location
Elastic cartilage			
1. Chondrocytes in lacunae	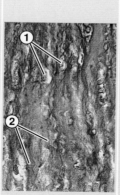	1. Produce and maintain ECM	1. Throughout cartilage
2. ECM: Composed of abundant elastic fibers and hair-like, branching strands in various orientations		2. Provide flexibility and elasticity	2. Throughout cartilage, in between chondrocytes
3. Perichondrium: Dense connective tissue		3. Protect and deliver vascular supply to the cartilage	3. Surrounding the outer surface of the cartilage
Fibrocartilage			
Firm, solid tissue that resembles dense connective tissue but contains:		Provide structural support and rigidity to resist compression and shearing forces and absorb shock	Pubic symphysis, annulus fibrosus of intervertebral discs, menisci
1. Chondrocytes in lacunae		1. Produce and maintain ECM	1. Throughout cartilage
2. ECM: Composed of abundant collagen fibers and thick, long strands often in one orientation No distinct perichondrium		2. Provide strength and flexibility	2. Throughout cartilage, in between chondrocytes

Additional Concepts

- **Cartilage is avascular:** Despite being a connective tissue, cartilage is avascular and, hence, relies on diffusion of nutrients from the vessels in the perichondrium or other surrounding tissues. Avascularity of the cartilage also contributes to slow and limited ability to heal and repair itself when injury occurs.
- **Growth of cartilage:** Mainly occurs during embryonic, fetal development and childhood, slowly decreasing in adolescence. In adults, cartilage undergoes little to no growth.
  - **Appositional growth:** Chondroblasts in the perichondrium produce cartilaginous matrix and thicken the cartilage from the periphery. Once the chondroblasts become encased in the matrix they produced, they become chondrocytes.
  - **Interstitial growth:** Chondrocytes in the middle of the cartilage divide, and then each daughter cell starts secreting its own cartilaginous matrix around itself, eventually becoming separated from each other by the newly produced cartilage matrix.
  - **Isogenous group:** A group of chondrocytes that arose from a single chondrocyte during interstitial growth. In the early stage, isogenous groups of chondrocytes can be identified by their close proximity to each other or sometimes by a number of chondrocytes sharing a single lacuna.

SUPPORTING CONNECTIVE TISSUE: GENERAL FEATURES OF THE BONE		
Structure	**Function**	**Location**
Cells		
1. Osteoprogenitors: Pool of mesenchymal stem cells, stellate to squamous morphology, difficult to identify on regular stain		1. Give rise to osteoblasts; with appropriate stimuli, may differentiate into other types of connective tissue cells	1. Mesenchyme, innermost layer of periosteum; endosteum; bone marrow

(continued)

SUPPORTING CONNECTIVE TISSUE: GENERAL FEATURES OF THE BONE (continued)

Structure		Function	Location
Cells			
2. Osteoblasts: a. Active: Cuboidal to columnar with baso-philic cyto-plasm and euchro-matic nuclei and distinct nucleoli b. Inactive: Squamous, difficult to identify	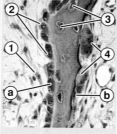	2. Secrete osteoid (type I col-lagen and bony matrix proteins) that calcifies	2. Innermost layer of periosteum; endosteum; usually in contact with the newly forming bone tissue
3. Osteocytes: Osteoblasts encased in calci-fied matrix mature and become osteocytes. Dendritic morphology	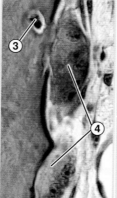	3. Maintain bony matrix; mechano-transduction	3. Main cell body in lacunae, cell processes in canaliculi
4. Osteoclasts: Large, mul-tinucleated macrophage derivative		4. Resorb bone tissue	4. Resorption bay (Howship lacunae): A concave depression on bone surface, scattered throughout endosteum and perios-teum

Structure	Function	Location
Coverings		
1. Periosteum: Dense connective tissue	1. Deliver neurovascular supply to the bone, allow tight attachment of the muscles and other structures to the bone	1. Outer surfaces of most compact bones
2. Endosteum: Resembles simple squamous epithelium composed of inactive osteoblasts, osteoprogenitors, and osteoclasts	2. Source of new osteoblasts and osteocytes	2. Inner surfaces of compact bones, canals; outer surfaces of all sponge bones

SUPPORTING CONNECTIVE TISSUE: BONE

Structure	Function	Location
Macroscopic features		
Specialized cells embedded in calcified ECM	Weight bearing, structural support, mineral storage	Long, short, flat, irregular bones of the body
1. Compact bone	1. Mechanical support, protection, weight transfer, mineral storage	1. Outer surfaces of the bones
2. Sponge bone	2. Weight transfer, quick mineral turnover	2. Inner portion of the bones

(continued)

SUPPORTING CONNECTIVE TISSUE: BONE (continued)

Structure		Function	Location
Macroscopic features			
3. Marrow space	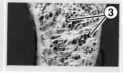	3. Site of blood formation and fat storage, lighten the weight of the bone	3. Spaces in between the sponge bone trabeculae
Compact (dense) bone			
Dense outer portions of the bone composed of:		Weight bearing, weight transfer, protection, site for muscle attachment	Peripheries of most bone; thicker in the diaphysis of long bones
1. Haversian system (osteons): Cylindrical structural units	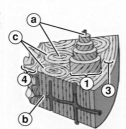	1. Bear and transfer weight in its long axis	1. Throughout compact bone, oriented parallel to the long axis of the bone or in the direction of applied force
a. Central/ Haversian canal: Central channel for vessels and nerves	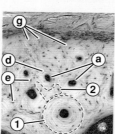	a. Conduct vessels and nerves throughout the length of the osteon	a. Center of each osteon
b. Perforating/ Volkmann canal: Channel that runs perpendicular to the long axis of osteon		b. Deliver vessels and nerves throughout the thickness of the compact bone	b. Varies, run perpendicular to the long axis of osteon

Structure		Function	Location
Compact (dense) bone			
c. Concentric lamellae: Concentric layers of bony matrix with collagen fibers in each layer running in opposite direction		c. Layered arrangements and fiber orientation allow optimal weight bearing and even weight transfer	c. Rings of bony matrix in each osteon
d. Cement line: Darker-staining line		d. Demark the outer limits of each osteon	d. Outer boundary of each osteon
e. Osteocytes in lacunae: Small openings/dots between the layers of concentric lamellae		e. Monitor and maintain the ECM	e. Wedged in between concentric and interstitial lamellae
f. Canaliculi: Short, narrow, hair-like channels		f. Conduct osteocyte processes, allow them to make physical and chemical contact via adhesions and gap junctions	f. Radiate from each lacuna and often run the width of each lamella
2. Interstitial lamellae: Noncylindrical layers of bony matrix		2. Fill the gap between osteons; weight bearing and transferring: Remnant of remodeled osteon	2. In between osteons

(continued)

SUPPORTING CONNECTIVE TISSUE: BONE (continued)

Structure	Function	Location

Compact (dense) bone

3. Outer circumferential lamellae: Several layers of bony matrix on the outer most side of the compact bone

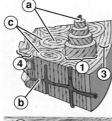

3. Bind the osteons from the outside, site of attachment for periosteum

3. Outermost layer of the compact bone

g. Sharpey fibers: Thick, ropy bundles of collagen type I fibers extending from periosteum into the compact bone

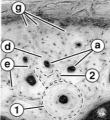

g. Tightly anchor periosteum to the compact bone

g. Extend from periosteum into the outer concentric lamellae and often deeper into the peripheral osteons

4. Inner circumferential lamellae: Several layers of bony matrix on the inside of the compact bone

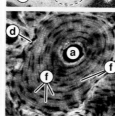

4. Bind the osteons from the inside, site of attachment for endosteum

4. Innermost layer of the compact bone

Sponge (cancellous/medullary) bone

Network of thin plates or branches of bony tissues with spaces in between:		Some role in weight transfer, reduce the weight of the bones, provide large surface area for bone resorption and formation	Center of diaphysis and epiphysis of long bones and center of most bones

Structure		Function	Location
Sponge (cancellous/medullary) bone			
1. Trabeculae (bony spicule): Small, thin, short bony tissues. In adults, bony matrix is lamellar (layered). No osteons		1. Collectively allow weight transfer, source of quick bone absorption and formation	1. Throughout central portion of most bones
2. Osteocytes in lacunae: Small openings/dots		2. Monitor and maintain bony matrix	2. Throughout trabeculae, in between bony matrix layers
3. Canaliculi: Short, narrow, hair-like channels		3. Conduct osteocyte processes, allow them to make physical and chemical contact via adhesion and gap junctions	3. Radiate from each lacuna and often run the width of each lamella
4. Endosteum:		4. Source of osteoprogenitors, osteoblasts, and osteoclasts	4. Inner surfaces of compact bones, canals; outer surfaces of all sponge bones
a. Inactive: Thin, delicate layer composed mostly of inactive osteoblasts, resembling simple squamous epithelium		a. Monitor and maintain bony matrix	a. Most adults

(continued)

SUPPORTING CONNECTIVE TISSUE: BONE (continued)

Structure		Function	Location
b. Active: Composed mostly of active osteoblasts, resemble simple cuboidal to columnar epithelium	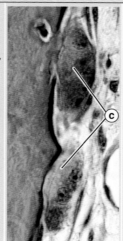	b. Build bone tissue	b. Embryos, infants, and young children
c. Osteoclasts: Large, multinucleated cells		c. Resorb bone tissue	c. Scattered throughout endosteum

Marrow cavity (space)

Space between trabeculae of the sponge bone filled with:		Lighten the bone	
1. Red marrow: Hematopoietic tissue	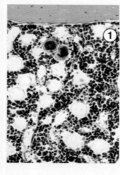	1. Blood cell production	1. Most marrow cavities in infants and young children. Marrow cavities of flat bones and vertebrae in adults
2. Yellow marrow: Unilocular adipose tissue		2. Lipid storage	2. Most marrow cavities of long bones in adults

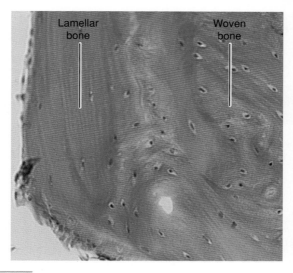

Figure 3-1. Histology of woven versus lamellar bone. (From Cui D. *Atlas of Histology*. Baltimore: Lippincott Williams & Wilkins, 2009:92.)

Additional Concepts

- **Woven versus lamellar bone:** Woven bone forms first during development, then is remodeled into lamellar bone (FIG. 3-1).
  - **Woven (primary, immature) bone:** First bone tissue that forms during ossification process. Collagen fibers are unorganized; osteocytes in lacunae are randomly scattered throughout bony matrix. Most compact and sponge bone in embryo and fetus initially forms as woven bone. In adults, woven bone is found in limited areas such as the site of healing bone and the alveolar processes of the maxilla and mandible.
  - **Lamellar (secondary, mature) bone:** Bone tissue that forms through remodeling of the woven bone. Collagen fibers are well organized; osteocytes in lacunae are regularly arranged and spaced throughout bony matrix, in between layers of bony matrix. Found in most adult compact and sponge bones.
- **Parathyroid hormone (PTH) versus calcitonin:** Two major hormones that regulate bone remodeling and blood calcium level (FIG. 3-2).

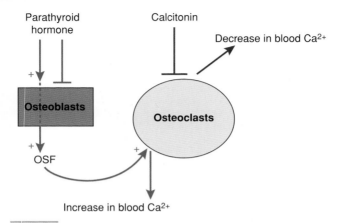

Figure 3-2. Hormonal regulation of bone remodeling and blood calcium level. (Asset provided by Lisa M.J. Lee, PhD. University of Colorado School of Medicine.)

- **PTH:** Is released by the parathyroid glands, inhibits osteoblasts from producing bony matrix, and stimulates its osteoclast-stimulating factor (OSF) secretion, which increases bone reabsorption by the osteoclasts, ultimately increasing the blood calcium level.
- **Calcitonin:** Is released by the parafollicular cells of the thyroid and inhibits osteoclasts, thus reducing bone reabsorption and ultimately decreasing blood calcium level.
- **Membranous versus endochondral ossification**
  - **Membranous (intramembranous) ossification:** Bone formation within the mesenchyme. Some of the mesenchymal cells aggregate, differentiate into osteoprogenitor cells, and give rise to osteoblasts. Osteoblasts produce bony matrix and become encased in it and become osteocytes. Newly formed bone matrices interconnect and remodel to form the compact and sponge bones of the flat bones and portions of irregular bones.
  - **Endochondral ossification:** Bone formation from the cartilage mold. Hyaline cartilage model of the bone forms first from the mesenchyme, which is then replaced by the bone tissue. Most long bones that need to lengthen rapidly form this way due to the ability of hyaline cartilage to form quickly without requiring a direct blood supply. As the cartilage model grows, a bone collar forms around the future diaphysis and blood vessels

grow into the center of the diaphysis to deliver osteoprogenitor cells that establish the primary ossification center. This process occurs in each epiphysis to establish the secondary ossification centers. At the junction between the primary and secondary ossification centers, a disc of hyaline cartilage remains as the growth plate (epiphyseal plate) that continues to produce hyaline cartilage. The rate of the hyaline cartilage replacement with bone tissue increases in adolescence until the entire growth plate becomes calcified, at which point the bone can no longer lengthen.

Clinical Significance

- **Osteoporosis:** Systemic skeletal disease of low bone density and increased susceptibility to fractures and skeletal deformity resulting from imbalance in bone building and reabsorption and/or insufficient calcium and other minerals in diet.
- **Rickets:** Insufficient calcification of bone tissues in children and adolescents due to insufficient calcium in diet or vitamin D deficiency. Skeletal deformity such as bowing of the long bones may occur in severe cases.

HISTOLOGIC LOOK-A-LIKES

	Hyaline Cartilage	Elastic Cartilage	Fibrocartilage
Fibers	Type II collagen, not obvious	Thin, branching elastic fibers in various orientations	Thick, long, rope-like bundles of collagen type I fibers often run in parallel
ECM	Glassy, homogenous appearance	Appears "busy" due to abundant elastic fibers that seem to outline many lacunae	Mixture of dense connective tissue and hyaline cartilage
Chondrocytes in lacunae	Relatively well (and evenly) spaced out	Closer to each other with thin bundle of elastic fibers running in between	Smaller in size; often several chondrocytes are grouped together in between bundles of collagen fibers

Once lacunae are observed, the tissue can only be cartilage or bone. In the absence of lamellar organization of the ECM and canaliculi, the tissue can only be one of the three cartilages.

Muscle Tissues | 4

INTRODUCTION

Muscle tissues are relatively cell dense, but their unique organization, specialized cell morphology, and stromal content allow effective identification and classification. Muscle tissues are specialized to contract and relax, producing movements of the body and organs.

MUSCLE TISSUES

THREE TYPES OF MUSCLE TISSUES		
Structure	**Function**	**Location**
Skeletal muscle		
1. Composed of long, striated, multinucleated muscle fibers; limited ability to renew	1. Production of major movements of the body	1. All over the body; most are attached to the bones
Cardiac muscle		
2. Composed of short, striated, uninucleate cardiomyocytes with branched cytoplasm, firmly attached to each other via intercalated discs; inability to renew	2. Coordinated contraction and relaxation fills and pumps blood	2. Heart

(continued)

THREE TYPES OF MUSCLE TISSUES (continued)		
Structure	**Function**	**Location**
Smooth muscle		
3. Composed of short, fusiform, uninucleate smooth muscle cells staggered in parallel; able to renew continually	3. Coordinated contraction of the visceral organs	3. Visceral organs, gastrointestinal tract (GI), blood vessels, exocrine glands, etc.

Additional Concepts

- Each muscle cell is also referred to as a muscle fiber.
- **Special terminologies for muscle fibers**
  - **Sarcolemma:** Muscle cell membrane
  - **Sarcoplasm:** Muscle cell cytoplasm
  - **Sarcoplasmic reticulum:** Muscle cell smooth endoplasmic reticulum (sER)
- Satellite cells in skeletal muscles have limited ability to proliferate and differentiate into skeletal muscle cells; as a result, extensive injury and destruction of muscle tissues cannot be fully repaired.
- Muscle-building exercises induce skeletal muscle hypertrophy (enlargement of each muscle fiber) rather than hyperplasia (increase in number of muscle fibers).

SKELETAL MUSCLE TISSUE		
Structure	**Function**	**Location**
Organization		
1. Skeletal muscle fiber: Striated, multinucleated muscle cell	1. Individual contractile cell	1. Throughout the muscle
2. Endomysium: Thin reticular fibers	2. Structural support for each cell and delivery of small vessels and nerves	2. Surround each muscle fiber

Structure		Function	Location
Organization			
3. Fascicle: A bundle of muscle fibers		3. Functional unit that works together	3. Throughout the muscle
4. Perimysium: Connective tissue		4. Bind each fascicle to help it function as a unit, deliver larger vessels and nerves	4. Surround each fascicle
5. Recognizable, named muscles: Formed by a collection of fascicles		5. Work in a coordinated manner to create movements	5. Throughout the body
6. Epimysium: Dense connective tissue		6. Sheath the muscle, help transmit contractile force of the muscle, deliver major vessels and nerves	6. Surround each muscle
Skeletal muscle cell (fiber)			
1. Myofibrils: Thin and long bundles that fill the muscle fiber 2. Sarcomere: Contractile unit of the myofibril		1. Contractile structure as long as the muscle cell 2. Line up back to back to form a myofibril	1. Throughout sarcoplasm 2. Length of myofibril

(continued)

SKELETAL MUSCLE TISSUE (continued)

Structure	Function	Location

Skeletal muscle cell (fiber)

3. Myofilaments: Strands of protein polymers
   a. Thick filaments: Myosin
   b. Thin filaments: Actin

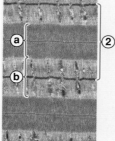
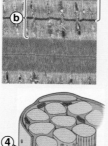

3. Interaction between thick and thin filaments produces contraction; overlap between the two filaments creates banding patterns (striations)

3. Within each sarcomere

4. Sarcoplasmic reticulum: Network of sER surrounds each myofibril
   c. Terminal cisterna: Dilated ring of sarcoplasmic reticulum

4. Store, release, and reuptake Ca^{2+}

4. Throughout sarcoplasm, surrounding each myofibril
   c. Between A and I bands

5. Transverse tubules (T tubules): Invagination of sarcoplasmic reticulum

5. Transmit membrane depolarization throughout sarcoplasm, trigger Ca^{2+} release from terminal cisternae

5. Travel through the muscle fiber at A–I junctions

Structure		Function	Location
Triad			
A unit of two terminal cisternae with a T tubule in the middle		Effective depolarization wave transmission and release of Ca^{2+}	A–I junctions
Striations			
Formed by the alternating thick and thin filaments			
1. A band: Dark band		1. Span of thick filaments; areas of overlap with thin filaments on either side	1. Middle portion of sarcomere
2. H band: Less dark band in the middle of A band		2. Portion of A band with only thick filaments	2. Middle portion of A band
3. M line: Faint, thin line in the middle of A band		3. Anchor thick filaments	3. Midline of A band
4. I band: Light band		4. Area with only thin filaments	4. Lateral portion spanning two sarcomeres
5. Z line (Z disc): Dense line in the middle of I band		5. Anchor thin filaments and mark the boundary of sarcomere	5. End margin of each sarcomere, midline of I band

(continued)

SKELETAL MUSCLE TISSUE (continued)		
Structure	**Function**	**Location**
Neuromuscular junction (motor end plate)		
Site of interaction between: 1. Motor axon terminal: Highly branched; contains numerous acetylcholine (ACh)-filled vesicles 2. Receptor region on sarcolemma: Shallow depression with many membrane folds (junctional folds) expressing cholinergic receptors for ACh		Usually in the middle of the muscle fiber but may vary
	1. In response to action potential, release ACh to the synaptic cleft 2. ACh receptors bind ACh and initiate membrane depolarization wave throughout muscle fiber.	

Additional Concepts

- **Motor unit:** A group of skeletal muscle fibers innervated by a single motor neuron that contract together
  - **Large motor unit:** A large group of muscle fibers innervated by a single motor neuron that generates a large contractile force but is relatively slow to respond as a whole. Includes postural muscles of the back, thighs, and buttocks
  - **Small motor unit:** A small group of muscle fibers innervated by a single motor neuron that generates fine, delicate movements fast. Includes extrinsic eye muscles and muscles that control the fingers
- **Sliding filament model:** Mechanism of contraction in which thin filaments slide on thick filaments toward the M line, shortening each sarcomere of myofibrils to produce contraction of each muscle fiber

- **Muscle contraction process:** Action potential travels down the axon → This triggers release of ACh at neuromuscular junction (NMJ) → ACh binds receptors on sarcolemma at NMJ → Sarcolemma depolarization wave travels through the rest of the cell and T tubules → Terminal cisternae release Ca^{2+} → Ca^{2+} allows interaction of myosin and actin → Adenosine triphosphate (ATP) is used to slide filaments on each other, which → shortens each sarcomere, which → shortens each myofibril → Muscle contraction is generated.

THREE TYPES OF SKELETAL MUSCLE FIBERS		
Structure	Function	Location
Type I (red, slow-twitch) fibers		
1. Small diameter; red appearance in vivo due to high myoglobin content; many mitochondria	1. Slow to contract but resistant to fatigue; undergo oxidative phosphorylation to produce maximum ATP	1. Postural muscles; large amount in muscles of endurance athletes
Type IIa (intermediate) fibers		
2. Medium-sized diameter; slightly red due to good amount of myoglobin; many mitochondria; glycogen storage	2. Faster to contract and fairly resistant to fatigue; generate ATP by both oxidative phosphorylation and glycolysis	2. Large amount in mid-distance runners and swimmers
Type IIb (white, fast-twitch) fibers		
3. Large diameter; light pink in vivo due to less myoglobin; fewer mitochondria; large glycogen storage	3. Fast to contract and prone to fatigue; generate ATP rapidly by anaerobic glycolysis. Lactic acid by-products cause fatigue	3. Extraocular muscles, muscles of the fingers; large amount in short-distance runners and weight lifters

MNEMONIC

The type and function of skeletal muscle fibers can be recalled by associating them with the famous fable **The Tortoise and the Hare**.

- Type I fibers are like the **tortoise**: Slow moving but steady, and they take first place (type I).
- Type IIb fibers are like the **hare**: Fast, but resting in the middle, and they come in last place (type IIb, the last of the three fibers).
- Type IIa fibers are in between the other two, chronologically. They come in the middle and, hence, are intermediate fibers.

Clinical Significance

- **Rigor mortis:** At the time of death, Ca^{2+} leaks out into sarcolemma → Actin and myosin interact → Due to lack of ATP, the interaction cannot be separated → This results in muscle rigidity.
- **Atrophy:** Decrease in muscle cell volume with the loss of myofibrils as the result of inactivity or loss of motor innervation
- **Myasthenia gravis:** Episodic and progressive muscle weakness commonly as the result of autoimmune antibody binding and blocking ACh receptors at neuromuscular junctions

CARDIAC MUSCLE TISSUE		
Structure	**Function**	**Location**
Cardiac muscle cell (cardiomyocyte)		
1. Single, oval nucleus	1. Regulate cardiomyocyte structure and function	1. Center of the cell
2. Striations: Same organization of bands as skeletal muscle cells	2. Sliding filaments generate contraction.	2. Throughout the cell
3. Glycogen storage: Clear-staining vesicles	3. Store energy	3. Throughout the cell, perinuclear area
4. Intercalated discs: Dark bands between cardiomyocytes	4. Create cardiomyocyte syncytium	4. In between cardiomyocytes

Structure	Function	Location
Cardiac muscle cell (cardiomyocyte)		
a. Transverse portion: Adhesion junctions and desmosomes	a. Adheres cardiomyocytes end to end	a. Portions of the disc perpendicular to long axis of the cell (filaments)
b. Lateral portion: Gap junctions	b. Transmission of macromolecules and ions between cells	b. Portions of the disc parallel to long axis of the cell (filaments)
5. Sarcoplasmic reticulum: Network of sER	5–6. Store, release, and reuptake Ca^{2+}	5. Throughout sarcoplasm
6. Terminal cisterna: Dilated portions of sarcoplasmic reticulum		6. At the level of Z lines
7. Transverse tubules (T tubules): Invagination of sarcoplasmic reticulum	7. Transmit membrane depolarization throughout sarcoplasm, trigger Ca^{2+} release from terminal cisternae	7. Travel through the muscle fiber at the level of Z lines
8. Diad: A unit of one terminal cisterna and a T tubule	8. Effective depolarization wave transmission and release of Ca^{2+}	8. Level of Z lines

Clinical Significance

- **Myocardial infarction (MI):** Injury and cell death at a region of the heart as a result of poor or blocked blood supply. Injured area is replaced by scar tissue rather than new cardiac cells due to their inability to proliferate.

SMOOTH MUSCLE TISSUE

Structure	Function	Location
Smooth muscle cell		
1. Single, elongated nucleus; may appear coiled in contracted cells	1. Regulate muscle cell structure and function	1. Center of the cell in longitudinal axis
2. Homogenous eosinophilic cytoplasm: No striations or bands	2. Contain organelles and contractile structures	2. Throughout the cell
3. Dense bodies: A group of proteins on the cytoplasmic side of sarcolemma	3. Attach and anchor thin filaments to sarcolemma	3. Scattered throughout the cytoplasmic side of sarcolemma
4. Gap junctions	4. Allow passage of macromolecules, ions between cells to function as a unit	4. Between cells

Clinical Significance

- **Leiomyoma:** Benign smooth muscle tumors often arising in the uterus; the most common neoplasm in women
- **Leiomyosarcoma:** Malignant smooth muscle tumors; 10% to 20% of soft tissue tumors

Additional Concepts

HISTOLOGIC LOOK-A-LIKES

Longitudinal Sections	Smooth Muscle	Dense Regular Connective Tissue	Nerve
Nuclei	Mixture of euchromatin and heterochromatin. Some are spiraled. Each is located within smooth muscle cells.	Very thin, heterochromatic nuclei of fibrocytes—seemingly in between thick collagen fibers	Oval, shorter, rounder nuclei are located in the periphery of the Schwann cells.
Cytoplasm	Relatively uniform in size and shape	Extremely thin, almost indiscernible	Appears segmental and rounded with a thin line (axon) running in the middle
Cellularity	Most dense	Least dense	Intermediate
Staining	Generally eosinophilic due to abundant cytoplasm	Intensely eosinophilic due to collagen fibers	Irregular staining pattern, mixture of thin lines (axon) and clear staining area in the vicinity

Neural Tissue | 5

INTRODUCTION

Neural tissue is one of the four basic tissue types composed mostly of cells, neurons forming the parenchyma, and diverse glial cells forming the stroma. Collectively, neural tissues form a complex chemical network throughout the body and allow it to sense and respond to stimuli and perform movements in a coordinated manner. Neural tissues are anatomically organized into the central nervous system (CNS), consisting of the brain and the spinal cord, and the peripheral nervous system (PNS), composed of all other neural tissues in the body. Functionally, neural tissues are divided into the somatic nervous system (SNS)—those under voluntary control—and the autonomic nervous system (ANS)—those under involuntary control. The autonomic nervous system is further divided into the sympathetic and parasympathetic nervous systems.

NEURAL TISSUE

NEURAL TISSUE COMPONENTS		
Structure	**Function**	**Location**
Neurons (neural cells)		
Structural and functional unit of the nervous system. Diverse in size and shape	Sense and respond to stimuli and initiate movements	Throughout the body
1. Cell body (perikaryon/soma): biggest portion of the neuron	1. Production of neurotransmitters, maintenance of neuron structural integrity	1. Depends on the type of neuron: One end of multipolar neuron, midportion of bipolar neuron, varying areas in unipolar neuron

(continued)

NEURAL TISSUE COMPONENTS (continued)

Structure	Function	Location
Neurons (neural cells)		
a. Nucleus: Large, round, euchromatic, distinct nucleolus	a. Regulation of transcription and neuron function	a. Central portion of the cell body
b. Nissl bodies: Stacks of rough endoplasmic reticulum (rER), observed as basophilic spots in cytoplasm	b. Translation, neurotransmitter production	b. Throughout the cell body
c. Axon hillock: Triangular, pale-staining area on cell body	c. Origination of axon	c. One pole of the cell body
2. Dendrites: Branched projections from cell body	2. Receiving information from other neurons or external environment and relaying it to cell body	2. Various points of the cell body
3. Axon: Single, often very long cellular projection from cell body	3. Transduction of action potential from the cell body to another neuron or to an effector cell, transport of vesicles and organelles between cell body and axon terminals	3. Long, single projection from the cell body

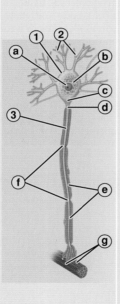

Structure	Function	Location
Neurons (neural cells)		
d. Initial segment: The first portion out of axon hillock	d. Action potential generation	d. Between the axon hillock and the first myelin sheath
e. Myelin sheath: Clear-staining glial cell (oligodendrocytes in CNS, Schwann cells in PNS) wrapping around axon at regular intervals	e. Axon insulation to ensure quicker transmission of action potential	e. Throughout the length of myelinated axons
f. Node of Ranvier: Unmyelinated segments of axon between myelin sheaths	f. Action potential propagation	f. In between two myelin sheaths
g. Axon terminals (boutons): Branched, dilated ends of an axon	g. Storage of neurotransmitter-filled vesicles, release and reuptake of neurotransmitters into and from the synaptic cleft	g. Ends of the axon, forming synapses with other neurons or effector cells/organs

(continued)

NEURAL TISSUE COMPONENTS (continued)

Structure		Function	Location
Three types of neurons based on morphology			

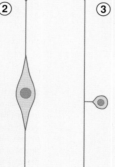

1. Multipolar neuron: Large cell body, many dendrites, a single axon
2. Bipolar neuron: Only two cellular processes from a fusiform cell body: One dendrite and one axon
3. Unipolar (pseudounipolar neuron): A spherical cell body that has a single cellular process that immediately branches into two long processes, one traveling to the CNS, the other to the periphery

1. Relay motor information or form a part of integrating network with other neurons
2. Relay special sensory information to the CNS
3. Relay sensory information from the periphery to the CNS

1. Numerous, found throughout neural tissue
2. Rare, found in special sensory organs such as retina and inner ear
3. Numerous, found throughout neural tissue. Collection of unipolar neuron cell bodies are found in spinal ganglia and cranial nerve ganglia.

Structure		Function	Location
Glial cells			
Group of non-conducting cells that together function as the supporting component of the neural tissue		Physical support, insulation of the neurons and synaptic clefts, repair of injured neurons, aid in metabolic exchange	Found throughout CNS and PNS
1. Astrocytes: Highly branched; indistinct cell boundaries; small, rounded nuclei with mixture of heterochromatin and euchromatin ("salt and pepper" pattern)		1. Providing physical support, participating in blood-brain barrier, taking part in metabolic exchange between neurons and vasculature	1. Only in the CNS; most numerous glial cells in the CNS
2. Oligodendrocytes: Indistinct cell boundaries; smallest, round, heterochromatic nuclei		2. Myelinating axons of the CNS; single cell can myelinate more than one axon.	2. Only in the CNS
3. Microglia: Indistinct cell boundaries; elongated, heterochromatic nuclei		3. Mediating neuroimmune reactions, phagocytosis of pathogens and cell debris	3. Only in the CNS

(continued)

NEURAL TISSUE COMPONENTS (continued)

Structure		Function	Location
Glial cells			
4. Ependymal cells: Cuboidal cells, clear cytoplasm, rounded nuclei, form simple cuboidal epithelia	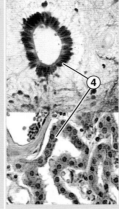	4. Lining the ventricles and central canal of the CNS, cerebrospinal fluid (CSF) production	4. Only in the CNS: Lining of the ventricles, choroid plexuses, lining of the central canal
5. Schwann cells: Each wrap around a single segment of an axon, oval to elongated nuclei in the cell periphery	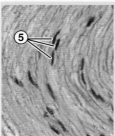	5. Myelinating axons in the PNS	5. Only in the PNS
6. Satellite cells: Indistinct cell boundaries; small, round, condensed nuclei	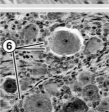	6. Supporting neuronal structures in the PNS	6. Only in the PNS; surrounding neuron cell bodies in ganglia

Structure	Function	Location
Meninges (coverings)		
Three layers of membranes that cover the CNS	Protect, anchor, and cushion brain and spinal cord	Surrounding brain and spinal cord
1. Dura mater: Dense connective tissue	1. Protecting and anchoring the brain and spinal cord	1. Outermost covering
a. Epidural space: Potential space above the dura	a. Potential space, normally closed off in the skull and filled with fatty tissue in the vertebral column	a. Between dura mater and skull in the head: between dura mater and vertebrae in the vertebral column
b. Subdural space: Potential space below the dura	b. Potential space, normally closed off	b. Between dura and arachnoid mater
2. Arachnoid mater: Delicate sheet of loose connective tissue	2. Providing nutritional support and limited protection	2. Deep to and in contact with the inside of dura mater
c. Arachnoid trabeculae: Web-like extensions of arachnoid	c. Providing limited structural support to the subarachnoid space and vasculature	c. Subarachnoid space

(continued)

NEURAL TISSUE COMPONENTS (continued)		
Structure	**Function**	**Location**
Meninges (coverings)		
d. Subarach-noid space: Actual space, filled with CSF	d. Providing cushion-ing mech-anism and vascular supply for brain and spinal cord	d. Between arachnoid and pia mater
3. Pia mater: Delicate and thin connec-tive tissue sheet	3. Lining the outermost layer of the CNS	3. Outermost layer of the brain and spinal cord

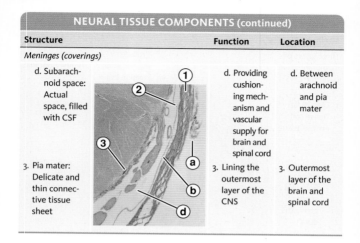

Additional Concepts

- **Three types of neurons based on function**
  - **Motor neurons:** Most are multipolar neurons that synapse with muscle cells to trigger contraction.
  - **Sensory neurons:** Most are unipolar neurons that carry sensory input from the periphery to the CNS. Cell bodies of the unipolar sensory neurons are accumulated in various ganglia throughout the body. Special sensory neurons of the retina and inner ear are bipolar neurons.
  - **Interneurons:** Multipolar neurons that integrate input from other neurons and relay the overall signal onto the next neuron.
- **Oligodendrocytes versus Schwann cells:** Both myelinate axons and perform similar functions; however, oligodendrocytes are only found in the CNS, whereas Schwann cells are only found in the PNS. A single Schwann cell can myelinate a small segment of a single axon in the PNS, whereas a single oligodendrocyte can myelinate small segments of more than one axon through its multiple cytoplasmic extensions.

CENTRAL NERVOUS SYSTEM: BRAIN		
Structure	Function	Location
Macroscopic features		
1. Cortex: Gray matter; abundant neuronal cell bodies cause gray hue.	1. Site of synapse; house neuronal cell bodies, dendrites, axons, and glia	1. Outer layer of the brain
2. Medulla: White matter; abundant axons, most of which are myelinated; give off glistening white hue	2. Conduction of neural impulse throughout axon fiber; house nuclei and tracts	2. Inner layer of the brain
3. Nuclei: Areas/ regions within medulla with a collection of neuronal cell bodies (gray matter)	3. Site of synapse and neural impulse integration	3. Scattered throughout medulla: Basal ganglia, lateral and medial geniculate nuclei, etc.
4. Tracts: Areas/ regions within medulla where white matter makes striations or distinct lines as a collection of axons travel together	4. House bundles of axons and associated glia	4. Throughout medulla: Corpus callosum, internal capsule, etc.

(continued)

CENTRAL NERVOUS SYSTEM: BRAIN (continued)

Structure		Function	Location

Microscopic features

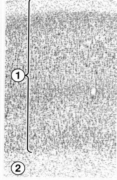

1. Cerebral cortex: Different types of neuronal cell bodies are organized into several recognizable layers; depending on the lobe or region of the brain, the pattern of the layers may differ.

   1. Site of synapse, integration of chemical signals and either inhibition or propagation of neural impulse

   1. Outer layer of the cerebrum, between pia mater and white matter

2. Cerebral medulla: Mostly myelinated axons and glial cells

   2. Conduction of neural impulse throughout axon fibers

   2. Inner layer of the cerebrum, deep to cortical gray matter

3. Cerebellar cortex: Gray matter composed of three distinct layers of neuronal cell bodies

   3. Site of synapse, integration of chemical signals and regulation of coordinated body movements and balance

   3. Outer, highly convoluted layer of the cerebellum

   a. Molecular layer: Relatively small neuronal cell bodies evenly distributed among glia

   a. Outermost layer, immediately below pia mater

Structure		Function	Location
Microscopic features			
b. Purkinje cell layer: Single layer of large pyramidal, multipolar neurons			b. Between molecular and granular layers
c. Granular layer: Densely distributed smallest neuronal cell bodies			c. Deepest layer of the cerebellar cortex
4. Cerebellar medulla: Mostly myelinated axons that form a thin, branched pattern of white matter (arbor vitae)		4. Conduction of neural impulse throughout axon fibers	4. Deep to cerebellar cortex

CENTRAL NERVOUS SYSTEM: SPINAL CORD

Structure		Function	Location
Microscopic features			
1. Cortex: White matter; axon bundles and glia forming various tracts		1. Conduction of neural impulse throughout axon fibers	1. Outer layer of the spinal cord, immediately below pia mater

(continued)

CENTRAL NERVOUS SYSTEM: SPINAL CORD (continued)

Structure		Function	Location
Microscopic features			

2. Medulla: Butterfly-shaped gray matter, neuronal cell bodies and glia

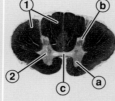

2. Site of synapse, integration of chemical signals and either inhibition or propagation of neural impulse

2. Inner, central portion of the spinal cord

a. Ventral horn: Anterior swelling of medulla containing cell bodies of motor neurons and glia

a. Neural integration, inhibition or propagation of action potential that results in muscle contraction

a. Anterior arms of the medulla

b. Dorsal horn: Cell bodies of interneurons; efferent axons of the sensory neurons and glia

b. Sensory neural integration, inhibition or propagation of action potential

b. Posterior arms of the medulla

c. Central canal: Narrow tubule filled with CSF and lined with ependymal cells

c. Contain small amount of CSF

c. Center of the medulla

PERIPHERAL NERVOUS SYSTEM		
Structure	**Function**	**Location**
Nerves		
Collection of axons (myelinated or nonmyelinated) outside of the CNS, surrounded and organized by connective tissue sheath	Conduct neural signals to and from the CNS	Throughout the body
1. Axons: Thin, long, delicate strands seen best in the middle of myelin sheaths	1. Conduct action potentials	1. Throughout the nerve
a. Myelinated axons: In longitudinal section, appear as chains of clear-staining area, each with an axon running in the middle. In cross section, appear as clear-staining circles, each with a central spot (axon)	a. Myelin sheath insulates the axons to allow faster conduction of action potential.	a. Throughout the nerve

(continued)

PERIPHERAL NERVOUS SYSTEM (continued)

Structure		Function	Location
Nerves			
b. Node of Ranvier: Portion of the myelinated axon, not covered by a Schwann cell, demarcated by a thin line and small indentation in between two myelin sheaths	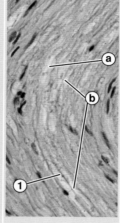	b. Propagates action potential at regular intervals throughout the length of the axon	b. On myelinated axons
c. Nonmyelinated axons: Collection of thread-like axons without abundant clear-staining areas. Streaks of darker-staining regions with crowded Schwann cell nuclei		c. Noninsulated axons conduct action potential at a slower rate	c. Throughout the nerve
Surrounded by:	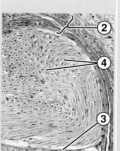		
2. Epineurium: Dense connective tissue around the entire nerve		2. Surround and protect the nerve, deliver vascular supply	2. Outermost layer of the nerve
3. Perineurium: Connective tissue around a bundle of axons (fascicles)		3. Surround a fascicle (bundle) of axons, deliver vascular supply	3. Extend from the epineurium into the nerve

Structure		Function	Location
Nerves			
4. Endoneurium: Delicate basement membrane around each axon or Schwann cell		4. Surround and support each axon and/or myelin sheath of an axon	4. In contact with axons and myelin sheaths
Ganglia			
Collection of neuronal cell bodies outside of the CNS		Regulate and maintain the neuronal cell integrity in the PNS	Throughout the body outside of the CNS
1. Spinal ganglia (dorsal root/ sensory ganglia)		1. Contain cell bodies of the sensory unipolar neurons	1. Bilateral swellings on either side of the spinal cord
a. Capsule: Dense connective tissue, continuation of the dura mater		a. Surround and protect the ganglia	a. Outermost layer
b. Unipolar neuronal cell bodies of varying size; arranged in clumps		b. Maintain and regulate neuron function	b. Throughout ganglia arranged in clumps
c. Satellite cells: Glial cells with indistinct cell body and small, round nuclei; resemble astrocytes		c. Support neurons in the PNS	c. Surrounding neuronal cell bodies and throughout ganglia
d. Axon bundles: Form strands that resemble tracts		d. Conduct action potential	d. Randomly traverse the ganglia

(continued)

PERIPHERAL NERVOUS SYSTEM (continued)

Structure		Function	Location

Ganglia

2. Sympathetic ganglia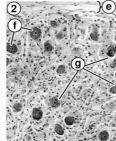

2. Contain cell bodies of the postsynaptic neuron cell bodies

2. In bilateral chain lateral to vertebral column

e. Capsule: Dense connective tissue

e. Surround and protect the ganglia

e. Outermost layer

f. Postsynaptic multipolar neuron cell bodies; evenly sized and distributed

f. Receive and integrate sympathetic signal

f. Throughout ganglia, evenly distributed

g. Satellite cells: Surround cell body but not as evenly positioned

g. Support neurons in the PNS

g. Throughout ganglia

3. Parasympathetic (enteric) ganglia: Small, pale-staining oval structures with no distinct capsule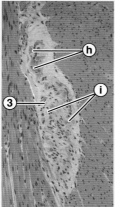

3. Contain cell bodies of the postsynaptic neurons

3. Close to and within visceral organs

h. Postsynaptic neuron cell bodies: Relatively large and triangular

h. Receive and integrate parasympathetic signal

h. Scattered throughout ganglia

Structure	Function	Location
Ganglia		
i. Satellite cells: Do not surround cell bodies at regular intervals	i. Support the neuron	i. Scattered randomly throughout ganglia

Additional Concepts

- **Synapse:** Site of communicational contact between two neurons or a neuron and an effector cell. A synapse is composed of a presynaptic axon terminal, a synaptic cleft, and a postsynaptic dendrite or effector cell (FIG. 5-1). When an action potential reaches the axon terminal, the membrane calcium channels open to allow the influx of Ca^{2+} into the axon terminal, triggering the secretory vesicles to fuse with the membrane and release the neurotransmitters into the synaptic cleft. Neurotransmitters then bind the receptors on the postsynaptic cell membrane and either initiate or inhibit the generation of action potential in the postsynaptic neuron.

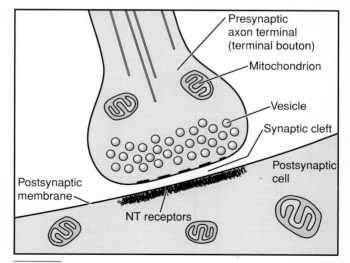

Figure 5-1. Synapse. (From Cui D. *Atlas of Histology with Functional and Clinical Correlations.* Baltimore: Lippincott Williams & Wilkins, 2009:119.)

- **Removal of neurotransmitters from the synaptic cleft:** Achieved by (1) the reuptake (endocytosis) by the presynaptic axon terminal, (2) degradation of neurotransmitters by the enzymes in the synaptic cleft, and (3) endocytosis and degradation by the postsynaptic cell. Without swift removal of the neurotransmitters, the postsynaptic cell may continue to be inhibited or continue to fire action potentials, resulting in unwanted effects downstream.
- **Blood-brain barrier:** Contains the following three components:
  - **Continuous capillaries:** Endothelial tight junctions create a seal that limits paracellular traffic. Gas and small lipid-soluble substances can pass through the cell, and select small molecules are transported through the endothelial cells. Endothelial cells in the nervous system express abundant receptors for essential molecules such as glucose, amino acids, and vitamins.
  - **Astrocyte end-foot processes** coat the outside of the capillaries and contribute to maintain endothelial cells and their tight junction integrity.
  - **Basement membrane** between the endothelium and the astrocyte foot processes
- **Unmyelinated axons** are still associated and supported by the oligodendrocytes in the CNS and by the Schwann cells in the PNS. More than one axon invaginates into nearby glial cells; thus, portions of the axons are embedded and surrounded by the glial cell membranes (Fig. 5-2).

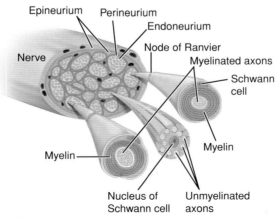

Figure 5-2. Myelinated and unmyelinated axons of the nerve. (From Ross M, Pawlina W. *Histology: A Text and Atlas.* 6th ed. Baltimore: Lippincott Williams & Wilkins, 2009:356.)

- **Response to neuronal injury in the PNS:** Portion of the axon distal to the injury degenerates (anterograde/Wallerian degeneration). Schwann cells surrounding the degenerating axons break down the myelin sheath, divide, and rearrange into a cellular column (band of Büngner). Macrophages clear the myelin debris. The injured neuron cell body undergoes chromatolysis, characterized by swelling, a reduction in Nissl bodies, and peripheral positioning of the nucleus. The regenerating axon branches into numerous sprouts (neurites). Once a neurite makes contact with a band of Büngner, it grows down its length and re-establishes contact with the postsynaptic cell. If neurites fail to make contact with the band of Büngner, the band eventually degenerates and reinnervation is not established (FIG. 5-3).

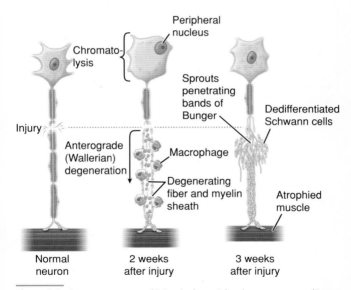

Figure 5-3. Response to neuronal injury in the peripheral nervous system. (From Ross M, Pawlina W. *Histology: A Text and Atlas.* 6th ed. Baltimore: Lippincott Williams & Wilkins, 2009:387.)

Clinical Significance

- **Pharmaceutical agents:** A number of pharmaceutical agents target the components of the synaptic cleft to either prolong or reduce the effects of neurotransmitters.
  - **Inhibitors of neurotransmitter reuptake:** Prolong the presence of neurotransmitters in the synaptic cleft, thus increasing the effects of neurotransmitters in the postsynaptic cells
  - **Inhibitors of enzymes that degrade neurotransmitters:** Increase the available pool of neurotransmitters, thus prolonging the effects of neurotransmitters in the postsynaptic cells

HISTOLOGIC LOOK-A-LIKES

	Dense Regular Connective Tissue	Nerve	Smooth Muscle
Cells	Flattened, thread-like fibrocyte nuclei are seen throughout, but are not abundant.	Oval nuclei of Schwann cells seen around the clear-staining myelin sheaths, and thread-like axon fibers observed in the middle	Looks much more cell dense with oval, sometimes spiraling nuclei in the middle of the cells and close to each other
Staining pattern	Intensely eosinophilic with thick bundles of collagen fibers dominating the visual field	Uneven staining with pale areas due to myelin sheaths and more eosinophilic areas where axons and Schwann cells are crowded	Relatively homogenous, basophilic staining pattern due to smooth muscle cell cytoplasm

Circulatory System | 6

INTRODUCTION

The circulatory system is composed of the heart and series of vessels that transport blood and lymph throughout the body. Blood is a specialized connective tissue composed of cells suspended in a large volume of fluid extracellular matrix. The four-chambered human heart is specialized to receive blood returning from the body and then to pump it to either the lungs or the rest of the body in a coordinated manner, with little to no backflow. Blood vascular histology varies depending on its function and location. The vessels close to the heart are designed to withstand large and repeatedly changing blood pressure and those much farther away are specialized to allow efficient exchange of gas and other molecules. The hydrostatic pressure and the composition of the blood within the vasculature play a critical role in maintaining fluid homeostasis throughout the body.

THE CIRCULATORY SYSTEM

BLOOD			
Structure		Function	Location
Composition			
Specialized connective tissue		Delivery of nutrients and O_2, transport of waste and CO_2, hormone delivery, facilitation of coagulation and immune response by delivery of white blood cells and platelets	Throughout the body within the heart and blood vessels

(continued)

BLOOD (continued)		
Structure	**Function**	**Location**

Composition

1. Plasma: Fluid extracellular matrix, 55% volume of blood	1. Functioning as solvent, buffering medium; maintaining osmotic pressure	1. Liquid supernatant
2. Formed elements: Cells and platelets, 45% volume of blood	2. Exchange of O_2, CO_2; participation in immune response and clotting	2. Sediment
a. Hematocrit: Majority of formed element, the volume of erythrocytes in a blood sample		a. Bottom layer
b. Buffy coat: 1% of blood volume, narrow, gray layer on top of hematocrit composed of leukocytes and platelets		b. On top of the hematocrit layer

Formed elements

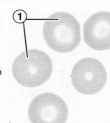

1. Red blood cells (erythrocytes): Red, biconcave, anucleate cells, 7.8 μm in diameter	1. Exchange of O_2 and CO_2	Suspended throughout plasma

Structure		Function	Location
Formed elements			
2. White blood cells: Nucleated cells of varying size and shape		2. Participation in immune surveillance and response	
a. Neutrophils: Lobed nuclei (three to four lobes), slightly granular cytoplasm		a. Responding to acute injury or infection, moving into the affected site, phagocytosis of pathogens or debris	
b. Lymphocytes: Small, spherical cells with spherical to slightly indented, heterochromatic nuclei; scant, clear cytoplasm		b. Responding to chronic injury or infection by engaging in adaptive immune response	
c. Monocytes: Larger cells; oval to kidney bean–shaped nuclei; larger, agranular cytoplasm		c. Responding to injury or infection by moving into the affected site and differentiating into macrophages	
d. Eosinophils: Bilobed nuclei, eosinophilic granule-filled cytoplasm		d. Responding to allergens, parasitic infections, and chronic inflammation	

(continued)

BLOOD (continued)		
Structure	Function	Location
Formed elements		
e. Basophils: Lobed nuclei, basophilic granule-filled cytoplasm	e. Releasing of vasoactive agents	
3. Platelets (thrombocytes): Small, anucleate cell fragments	3. Blood clot formation and repair of injury	

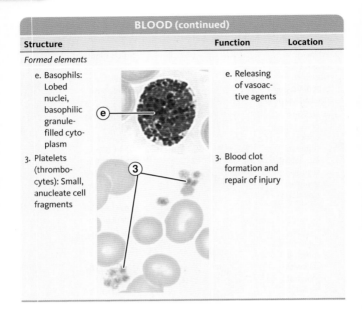

Additional Concepts

- **Hematocrit:** Volume of packed erythrocytes in a blood sample. Normal range is 39% to 50% in males and 35% to 45% in females.
- **Shape of the erythrocyte:** Maintained by a variety membrane proteins (Fig. 6-1).
  - **Integral membrane proteins:** Embedded within the phospholipid bilayer membrane and function as the sites of attachments for peripheral membrane proteins. The extracellular domains are glycosylated, which contributes to blood group antigen specification.
  - **Peripheral membrane proteins:** Associated with the inner surface of the phospholipid bilayer membrane that forms a meshwork that holds the unique biconcave shape of the erythrocytes while providing it with a level of flexibility.
- **Histologic ruler:** Due to uniform size and abundant presence throughout the body, erythrocytes serve as a useful marker for estimating relative size of the cells and other structures in a tissue.
- **Granulocytes versus agranulocytes**
  - Granulocytes contain specific granules in addition to lysosomes in the cytoplasm and include neutrophils, eosinophils, and basophils.

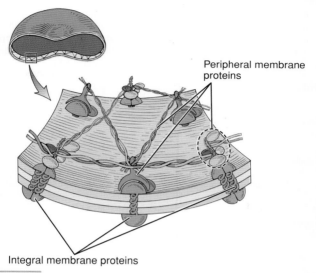

Peripheral membrane proteins

Integral membrane proteins

Figure 6-1. Proteins that maintain shape and function of erythrocytes. (From Ross MH, Pawlina W. *Histology: A Text and Atlas*. 6th ed. Baltimore: Lippincott Williams & Wilkins, 2009:272.)

- Agranulocytes do not have specific granules in the cytoplasm and include lymphocytes and monocytes. Lysosomes are present in agranulocytes; however, they do not present as particularly well-staining granules. Hence, the cells appear to be agranular.
- **Three types of lymphocytes:** B lymphocytes, T lymphocytes, and natural killer cells perform different functions in the immune system but are indistinguishable from each other on regular staining.

Clinical Significance

- **Anemia:** Reduced hematocrit. A variety of conditions may cause anemia such as internal or external bleeding or any condition that reduces erythropoiesis.
- **Sickle cell anemia:** Most common cause of sickle cell anemia is a single amino acid change from glutamic acid to valine in the β-globin subunit of hemoglobin. Under stressful conditions such as acute or chronic infection and increased oxygen demand, mutated hemoglobins coalesce and alter the shape of the red blood cells into sickle shape. Sickle cells are less flexible and hence

easily block narrow capillaries, causing tissue injury and necrosis downstream, which are also associated with a significant amount of pain. Sickle cells have shorter life spans than regular erythrocytes as they are easily trapped and destroyed in the spleen and other sites; hence, patients often present with anemia.

HISTOLOGIC LOOK-A-LIKES

	Lymphocytes	Monocytes
Size	Most lymphocytes are small and closer to the size of erythrocytes	Large cells
Nuclei	Appear more homogenously heterochromatic, usually spherical, may contain a small indentation	Appear slightly more "thready" with a mix of euchromatic and heterochromatic areas, often contain small to large indentations and may appear kidney bean shaped
Cytoplasm	Scant cytoplasm with clear to blue hue, form a thin ring around the nucleus	Good amount of cytoplasm, slightly more eosinophilic and dusty appearance

MNEMONIC

Never Let Monkeys Eat Bananas

This phrase corresponds to the types of white blood cells in peripheral blood, in order of most to least abundant:

Neutrophils > **L**ymphocytes > **M**onocytes > **E**osinophils > **B**asophils

HEART		
Structure	**Function**	**Location**
Macroscopic features		
1. Right atrium: Thin-walled chamber; smooth glistening lining on dorsal side; triangular auricle with pectinate muscles on lateral, anterior side	1. Receiving deoxygenated blood from the systemic circulation and pumping it to the right ventricle	1. Right upper chamber

Structure		Function	Location
Macroscopic features			
2. Left atrium: Thin-walled chamber with mostly smooth, glistening lining; thin, long auricle with pectinate muscles on anterior side		2. Receiving oxygenated blood from the lungs and channeling it to the left ventricle	2. Left upper chamber
3. Right ventricle: Relatively thin but muscular chamber, elaborate trabeculae carinae and papillary muscles		3. Receiving blood from the right atrium and pumping it to the lungs	3. Right lower chamber
4. Left ventricle: Thick muscular chamber, trabeculae carinae and papillary muscles		4. Receiving blood from the left atrium and pumping it to the rest of the body	4. Left lower chamber
5. Fibroskeleton: Dense connective tissue		5. Physically blocking transduction of action potential between atria and ventricles, anchoring cardiac muscles and valves	5. Between atria and ventricles, surrounding each of the four main entry and exit orifices
6. Valves: Fibrous flaps		6. Preventing regurgitation of blood during contraction	6. Within atrioventricular orifices

(continued)

HEART (continued)		
Structure	**Function**	**Location**

Microscopic features

1. Endocardium: Thin layer of connective tissue in contact with blood in the lumen

1. Lining and supporting the lumen of the heart

1. Innermost layer

a. Endothelium: Simple squamous epithelium

a. Lining the lumen; regulating permeability, blood flow; producing anticoagulants

a. In contact with blood

b. Subendocardial layer: Connective tissues, scattered smooth muscle cells

b. Cushioning and supporting endothelium

b. Deep to endothelium

c. Purkinje fibers: Modified cardiomyocytes

c. Conducting action potential

c. Within subendocardial layer

2. Myocardium: Cardiac muscle fibers

2. Contracting to pump blood throughout the body

2. Middle layer of the heart

3. Epicardium: Same as visceral layer of pericardium

3. Lining and supporting the outside of the heart

3. Outer layer of the heart

d. Mesothelium: Simple squamous epithelium

d. Production of serous fluid

d. Outermost layer, in contact with pericardial fluid

Structure	Function	Location
Microscopic features		
e. Subepicardial connective tissue: Loose and adipose connective tissues	e. Support, protection, insulation of the heart	e. Between mesothelium and myocardium

GENERAL ORGANIZATION OF BLOOD VESSELS

Structure	Function	Location
Tunica intima		
1. Endothelium: Simple squamous epithelium	1. Lining the lumen; regulation of permeability, blood flow; production of anticoagulants	1. Innermost layer, in contact with blood
2. Subendothelial layer: Loose connective tissue	2. Cushioning and supporting endothelium	2. Deep to endothelium
3. Internal elastic lamina: Thin layer of elastic fibers	3. Providing limited elasticity and structural support	3. Outermost layer of the tunica intima
Tunica media		
4. Smooth muscle layer: Varies in thickness and stromal elastic fiber content	4. Contracting to regulate blood pressure and volume of blood passing through	4. Between internal and external elastic lamellae

(continued)

GENERAL ORGANIZATION OF BLOOD VESSELS (continued)

Structure	Function	Location
Tunica media		
5. External elastic lamina: Thin layer of elastic fibers	5. Providing limited elasticity and structural support	5. Between smooth muscle layer and tunica adventitia
Tunica adventitia		
6. Adventitia layer: Connective tissue	6. Providing structural support, anchoring the vessel to the surrounding tissues	6. Outermost layer of vessels
7. Vasa vasorum: Small blood vessels	7. Delivery of vascular supply to the outer wall of the vessel	7. Throughout tunica adventitia

ARTERIES

Structure	Function	Location
Elastic (large) arteries		
1. Thick tunica intima: Relatively thick	1. Lining and protecting the lumen	Aorta and other large branches off of the aorta
2. Thick tunica media with abundant elastic fibers (elastic connective tissue)	2. Allowing distension and recoil of the vessel to accommodate repeated fluctuation of blood pressure, ensuring steady flow of blood	

Structure		Function	Location
Elastic (large) arteries			
3. Relatively thin tunica adventitia (one-quarter to one-half the thickness of tunica media) a. Abundant vasa vaso-rum: Small blood vessels * Indistinct internal and external elastic laminae		3. Providing support and protection a. Delivery of vascular supply to the outer wall	
Muscular arteries			
1. Thinner tunica intima a. Distinct internal elastic lamina 2. Thick tunica media: Mostly smooth muscle tissue b. Distinct external elastic lamina 3. Tunica adventitia approximately the same thickness as tunica media c. Vasa vaso-rum: Small blood vessels		1. Lining and protecting the lumen a. Providing elasticity and structural support to tunica intima 2. Contracting to maintain blood pressure b. Providing elasticity 3. Providing support and protection c. Delivery of vascular supply to the outer wall	Distal arteries: Include splenic, renal, supra-renal, radial, and ulnar arteries

(continued)

ARTERIES (continued)

Structure	Function	Location
Small arteries		

1. Thin tunica intima
 	
   a. Distinct internal elastic lamina
 	
 2. Tunica media with three to eight layers of smooth muscle cells
 	
 3. Thinner tunica adventitia
 * Indistinct external elastic lamina
	1. Lining and protecting the lumen
	
	   a. Providing elasticity and structural support
	
	 2. Regulating blood flow to arterioles and capillary beds
	
	 3. Support and protection
		Distal branching arteries feeding into small regions of the body or organ

Arterioles		
1. Thin tunica intima 2. Tunica media with one to two layers of smooth muscles 3. Thin tunica adventitia * No internal and external elastic laminae	1. Lining and protecting the lumen 2. Regulating blood flow to capillary beds 3. Support, protection, and anchoring	Immediately before capillary beds

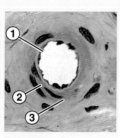

CAPILLARIES

Structure	Function	Location
Continuous capillaries		
Simple squamous epithelium lined with endothelial cells	Lining and protecting the lumen, tightly regulating transport of	Exocrine glands, muscle tissues, lungs, CNS, testes, thymic cortex

Structure		Function	Location
Continuous capillaries			
		molecules across the capillary wall	
1. Thin cytoplasm	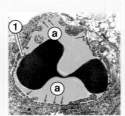	1. Ensuring fast exchange of gas and small, lipid-soluble molecules	1. Innermost layer in contact with blood
a. Pinocytic vesicles		a. Allowing transport of large volume of materials	a. Within endothelial cell cytoplasm
2. Flattened nuclei: Heterochromatic		2. Maintenance of endothelial cell	2. In endothelial cell, protruding out into the luminal space
3. Tight junctions between cells		3. Preventing paracellular exchange of materials	3. Between endothelial cells
Fenestrated capillaries			
Simple squamous epithelium lined with endothelial cells		Lining and protecting the lumen, transport of larger molecules across the capillary	Endocrine glands, intestinal tracts, kidneys
1. Thin cytoplasm		1. Aiding fast exchange of gas and small, lipid-soluble molecules	

(continued)

CAPILLARIES (continued)

Structure	Function	Location

Fenestrated capillaries

a. Fenestrae: Small holes throughout cytoplasm 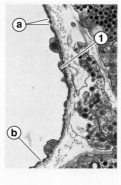	a. Forming channels across the capillary wall, allowing bigger molecule transport	
b. Diaphragm: Thin, non-cellular membrane across the openings of fenestrae	b. Unknown function	

Sinusoids (discontinuous capillaries)

Simple squamous epithelium lined with endothelial cells, large diameter	Lining and protecting the lumen while allowing large molecules and cells to move between the lumen and interstitium	Liver, spleen, bone marrow
1. Large openings between endothelial cells, partial to complete lack of basal lamina 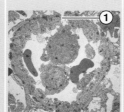	1. Transport of large molecules and cells between lumen and interstitium	

VEINS		
Structure	**Function**	**Location**
Venules		
Three tunics are thin and indistinct with diameter between 0.1 mm and less than 1 mm 1. Endothelium: Simple squamous epithelium 2. Thin tunica media: One to two layers of smooth muscles	Draining capillary beds, major response to vasoactive agents (histamine, serotonin)	Distal to capillary beds
Medium veins		
Diameter between 1 mm and 10 mm 1. Tunica intima: Endothelium, indistinct internal elastic lamina 2. Tunica media: Much thinner than medium arteries 3. Tunica adventitia: Relatively thick, over two times the thickness of tunica media 4. Valves: Thin connective tissue flaps lined with endothelium	Draining venules, preventing backflow of blood	Distal to venules

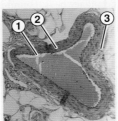

(continued)

VEINS (continued)		
Structure	Function	Location
Large veins		
Diameter greater than 10 mm 1. Tunica intima: Endothelium, small subendo- thelial tissue, indistinct internal elastic lamina 2. Tunica media: Relatively thin, several layers of smooth muscles 3. Tunica adventitia: Thickest of the three tunics	Draining medium venules and channeling blood toward the heart	Inferior vena cava, superior vena cava, hepatic portal vein, brachio- cephalic veins

Additional Concepts

- **Arteriovenous (AV) shunts:** Direct routes between arterioles and venules that bypass capillary beds. Found in the skin, erectile tissues, and areas of the gastrointestinal (GI) tract. When the AV shunts close, blood is forced to go through the capillaries before draining into the venules, thus slowing down the blood flow in a given area to promote exchange of molecules.
- **AV shunts in the skin:** Open in response to cold, allowing blood to run directly from arterioles to venules, bypassing the skin cap- illary beds in an effort to conserve heat. In response to heat, AV shunts close, forcing blood in the arterioles to flow through the capillary beds before draining into venules, thus allowing heat to be released from the surface of the body.
- **Pericytes:** Supportive cells that surround the outside of the capil- laries, arterioles, and venules. In addition to helping endothelial cells to maintain their function and integrity, pericytes possess the ability to contract and regulate flow of blood through the capillaries or venules.

Clinical Significance

- **Ischemic cardiomyopathy:** Most commonly caused by athero- sclerosis in which the coronary arteries become stenotic due to progressively thickening atheromatous plagues, resulting in an insufficient oxygen delivery to a region of the heart supported by the vessel.

- **Myocardial infarction:** Cardiac muscle cell death resulting from the lack of blood supply to a region of the heart, commonly due to near 100% stenotic coronary artery.
- **Atherosclerosis:** Accumulation of lipid and thickening of the tunica intima that eventually leads to stenosis of the artery. Atherosclerotic tissue weakens the arterial wall and may cause damage to the endothelium, making it susceptible to formation of thrombosis.
- **Deep vein thrombosis (DVT):** Blood clot formation most often in the deep veins of lower limbs associated with prolonged immobility and subsequent pooling of the stagnant blood in a vein. Once dislodged, the clot becomes an embolus and can be life-threatening when it travels through the circulatory system and gets lodged in other sites, commonly the pulmonary arteries.

Lymphatic System | 7

INTRODUCTION

The lymphatic system is composed of groups of cells, tissues, and organs that monitor the body for harmful substances and combat to eliminate them. Leukocytes, particularly lymphocytes, make up the parenchyma of the lymphoid system and are found in diffuse lymphoid tissues, lymphoid nodules, and lymphoid organs. Lymphoid organs are composed of lymphoid tissues surrounded by a connective tissue capsule. Lymphatic vessels allow communication among lymphatic structures and with the blood vascular system. Due to their important immunologic functions, structures of the lymphoid system are found throughout the body but are more prominent along the mucosa and at key points between the limbs and the trunk.

THE LYMPHATIC SYSTEM

LYMPHOID TISSUES		
Structure	Function	Location
Diffuse lymphoid tissue		
1. Relatively high concentration of leukocytes (primarily lymphocytes, plasma cells, eosinophils, and macrophages) evenly distributed in loose connective tissue matrix	1. Protection of the body from pathogens and initiation of immune response	1. Lamina propria of the gastrointestinal (GI), respiratory, and urinary tract mucosa; dispersed throughout lymphoid organs

(continued)

LYMPHOID TISSUES (continued)		
Structure	**Function**	**Location**
Lymphoid nodules (follicles)		
2. Dense aggregate of mostly B lymphocytes. When activated by antigens, lymphoid nodules produce antibodies	2. Protection of the body from pathogens and initiation of immune response	2. Lamina propria of the GI, respiratory, and urinary tract mucosa; dispersed throughout lymphoid organs; most prominent in tonsils, Peyer patches, and appendix
3. Germinal center: Lighter staining central area	3. Site of lymphocyte proliferation, plasma cell differentiation, and antibody production	3. In the center of activated lymphoid nodules
4. Mantle zone (corona): Ring of densely basophilic area	4. Composed of newly formed lymphocytes	4. Surround the germinal center

Additional Concepts

- **MALT (mucosa-associated lymphoid tissue):** Diffuses lymphoid tissues and lymphoid nodules that are closely associated with the mucosa.
  - **GALT (gut-associated lymphoid tissue):** The MALT in the GI tract mucosa.
  - **BALT (bronchus-associated lymphoid tissue):** The MALT in the respiratory tract mucosa.
- Tonsils are an example of GALT; however, because they exhibit a partial connective tissue capsule, tonsils are considered to be lymphoid organs.

TONSILS

Structure		Function	Location
Palatine tonsils (tonsils)			
Paired, dense collections of lymphoid tissues that contain:		Immune function at the entrance of the oropharynx	Either side of the oropharynx between palatopharyngeal and palatoglossal arches
1. Nonkeratinized stratified squamous epithelium		1. Form the protective mucosal lining	1. Pharyngeal surface of the tonsil
2. Crypts: Deep invaginations of lining epithelium with lymphocyte infiltrate		2. Increase surface area for contact between the oropharyngeal content and the immune cells	2. Extend into tonsillar parenchyma
3. Incomplete connective tissue capsule		3. Separate tonsils from underlying connective tissue and wall them off in the event of infection	3. Between the tonsil and underlying connective tissue
4. Diffuse lymphoid tissue		4–5. Immune function	4. Throughout tonsillar parenchyma
5. Numerous lymphoid nodules, many with prominent:			5. Throughout tonsillar parenchyma

(continued)

TONSILS (continued)		
Structure	**Function**	**Location**
Palatine tonsils (tonsils)		
a. Germinal centers b. Mantle zones (corona)		a. In the center of activated lymphoid nodules b. Peripheral margins of germinal centers
Pharyngeal tonsil (adenoid)		
Unpaired collection of lymphoid tissue that contains:	Immune function on the roof of the nasopharynx	Roof of the nasopharynx
1. Ciliated pseudostratified columnar epithelial lining	1. Form the mucosal lining	1. Pharyngeal surface
2. Incomplete connective tissue capsule	2. Separate the tonsil from underlying connective tissue and wall it off in the event of infection	2. Between the tonsil and underlying connective tissue
3. Numerous lymphoid nodules 4. Diffuse lymphoid tissue	3–4. Immune function	3–4. Throughout tonsillar parenchyma
Lingual tonsil		
Collection of lymphoid tissue:		Surface of the posterior third of the tongue
1. Nonkeratinized stratified squamous epithelium	1. Form the mucosal lining	1. Pharyngeal surface

Structure	Function	Location
Lingual tonsil		
2. Crypts: Wide invagination of lining epithelium	2. Increase surface area for contact between oropharyngeal content and immune cells	2. Extend into tonsillar parenchyma
3. Incomplete connective tissue capsule	3. Separate the tonsil from connective tissue	3. Between the tonsil and underlying connective tissue
4. Numerous lymphoid nodules and diffuse lymphoid tissue	4. Immune function	4. Throughout tonsillar parenchyma

HISTOLOGIC LOOK-A-LIKES

Although all three tonsils exhibit similar parenchymal histology of diffuse lymphoid tissue and lymphoid nodules, other structural features help distinguish the three.

	Palatine Tonsils	Pharyngeal Tonsils	Lingual Tonsils
Mucosal epithelium	Nonkeratinized stratified squamous epithelium	Ciliated pseudostratified columnar epithelium	Nonkeratinized stratified squamous epithelium
Crypts	Deep, branched, and numerous	None	Wide, short, and not branched

Clinical Significance

- **Tonsillitis:** Inflammation of the tonsils as the result of bacterial or viral infection. Red, swollen palatine tonsils with purulent exudates (pus) are easily observed when the patient opens the mouth and the tongue is depressed. Patients present with sore throat, pain, fever, and dysphagia. In severe cases, the infection may extend to involve the pharynx, larynx, and auditory tube.

LYMPH NODES

Structure	Function	Location
Macroscopic features		
Numerous oval structures of varying size throughout the body	Filtration of lymph	Found throughout the body along the lymphatic vessels; more numerous in axilla, groin, neck, and mesenteries
1. Convex side	1. Afferent lymphatic vessels enter	1. Portion with convex contour
2. Hilum: Indented area	2. Efferent lymphatic exit and blood vessels and nerves exit and enter	2. Concave area
3. Capsule with trabeculae: Dense connective tissue	3. Structural support	3. Superficial-most protective structure and its extensions into the lymphatic tissue
Microscopic features		
4. Outer (superficial/ nodular) cortex: Lymphoid nodules composed of mostly B lymphocytes	4. Screen the lymph for antigens, differentiate into plasma cells, and produce antibodies upon contact with an antigen	4. Deep to capsule
5. Inner (deep/ para-) cortex: Diffuse lymphoid tissue composed of mostly T lymphocytes	5. T cells interact with antigen-presenting cells	5. Between the outer cortex and the medulla

Structure	Function	Location
Microscopic features		
6. Medulla composed of:	6. Continued filtration and collection of lymph	6. Center of the lymph node
a. Medullary cords: Denser collections of B cells, plasma cells, macrophages, and reticular cells	a. Phagocytosis, antibody production	a. Scattered throughout medulla
b. Medullary sinuses: Lymphatic channels between the cords	b. Lymph flow and collection	b. In between medullary cords

Additional Concepts

- **Lymph:** Excess interstitial fluid that is collected and transported to blood circulatory system. Along the way, lymph is filtered by several lymph nodes for antigens or other potentially harmful particles or cells.
- **Flow of lymph through a lymph node:** Afferent lymphatic vessel → subcapsular (cortical) sinus → peritrabecular (trabecular) sinus → medullary sinus → efferent lymphatic vessel (FIG. 7-1).

Clinical Significance

- **Lymphadenitis:** Reactive, inflammatory enlargement of lymph nodes when lymphocytes respond to antigens by proliferating, forming germinal centers and producing antibodies. Enlarged lymph nodes are commonly referred to as swollen glands and can be observed or palpated in the neck of a patient with oropharyngeal infection or in the axilla or groin of a patient with an infection in the extremity.
- **Sentinel node:** The first lymph node or a group of lymph nodes that the lymph from certain regions of the body passes through.
- **Sentinel node biopsy:** Procedure in which sentinel nodes are removed to determine the presence of metastatic tumor cells to

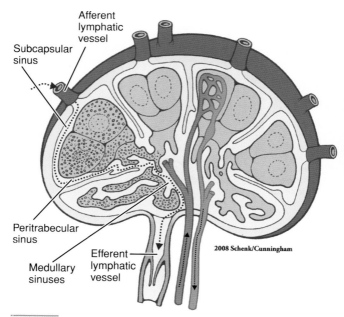

Afferent lymphatic vessel

Subcapsular sinus

Peritrabecular sinus

Medullary sinuses

Efferent lymphatic vessel

2008 Schenk/Cunningham

Figure 7-1. Flow of lymph through a lymph node. (From Cui D. *Atlas of Histology with Functional and Clinical Correlations.* Baltimore: Lippincott Williams & Wilkins, 2009:119.)

stage certain types of cancer. To identify sentinel nodes, surgeons inject dye or radioactive fluid into the tumor or its surrounding area then trace its path to find and biopsy the nodes.

THYMUS		
Structure	**Function**	**Location**
Macroscopic features		
Bilobed lymphoid organ:	Differentiation and maturation of T lymphocytes	Superior anterior mediastinum
1. Dense connective tissue capsule	1. Protection, outer boundary of the organ	1. Externalmost surface of the organ

Structure		Function	Location
Macroscopic features			
2. Trabeculae: Dense connective tissue extensions from the capsule into the parenchyma	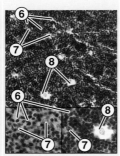	2. Form septa that separate thymic lobules, carry vessels and nerves	2. Extend into the parenchyma from the capsule
3. Cortex: Cell-dense, basophilic staining region		3. T-cell selection and maturation	3. Deep to the capsule
4. Medulla: Lighter-staining region		4. T-cell selection, maturation, storage, and release into circulation	4. Central region of the organ
5. Thymic (Hassall) corpuscles: Eosinophilic, spherical structures with concentric layers		5. Unclear	5. Scattered in the medulla
Microscopic features			
Cortex composed of:			
6. Thymocytes: Small, basophilic developing T cells		6. Undergoing selection and maturation	6–8. Throughout cortex and medulla
7. Epithelioreticular cells (types I, II, III): Stellate cells with larger, lighter-staining nuclei		7. Form architectural framework, contribute to thymic-blood barrier, participate in T-cell selection	
8. Macrophages: Clear-staining cytoplasm		8. Phagocytose unselected thymocytes	

(continued)

THYMUS (continued)		
Structure	Function	Location

Microscopic features

Medulla composed of more epithelioreticular cells (types IV, V, VI) and loosely packed, mature T cells and:

5. Thymic (Hassall) corpuscles: Concentric bundles of epithelioreticular cells

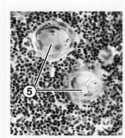

Additional Concepts

- **Blood-thymic barrier:** Composed of continuous capillaries and epithelioreticular cells that form a physical barrier between the thymocytes and blood to protect the developing thymocytes from antigen exposure, which can lead to compromised immune function.
- **Epithelioreticular cells versus reticular cells:** Two different groups of cells in terms of embryonic origin, morphology, and function. Due to both cells' involvement in the lymphoid system and possession of "reticular" in the name, students often confuse the two.
  - **Epithelioreticular cells:** Epithelioid in shape (broad, large cytoplasm), play a role in T-cell development, and only found in the thymus.
  - **Reticular cells:** Fibrocyte-like cells with thin, spindle-shaped morphology that produce reticular fibers in most lymphoid organs including the thymus.

SPLEEN		
Structure	**Function**	**Location**
Macroscopic features		
Single, fist-sized lymphoid organ:	Filtration, clearance of microorganisms, antigens from blood. Production of antibodies, removal of abnormal erythrocytes, hematopoiesis	Upper left quadrant in peritoneal cavity at 9–12 rib level
1. White pulps: Cell-dense, gray, nodular areas	1. Filter and monitor blood, produce antibodies when activated by an antigen	1–2. Throughout spleen
2. Red pulps: Softer, red, less cell-dense areas	2. Filter blood, destroy damaged or altered erythrocytes	
3. Capsule: Dense connective tissue	3. Protection and coverage	3. Surrounds the spleen
4. Trabeculae: Dense connective tissue	4. Structural support and delivery of vessels	4. Extensions of the capsular tissue into the parenchyma
Microscopic features		
White pulps:		
5. Lymphoid nodules; mostly B cells with or without germinal centers	5. Screen blood for antigens and produce plasma cells and antibodies	5. Throughout the organ

(continued)

SPLEEN (continued)		
Structure	**Function**	**Location**

Microscopic features

6. Germinal center: Lighter-staining area	6. B-cell proliferation, differentiation to plasma cells and antibody production	6. Center of lymphoid nodule

7. Central artery: Branch of splenic artery	7. Deliver blood to white and red pulps	7. Periphery of a white pulp lymphoid nodule
8. Periarterial lymphatic sheath (PALS): Aggregate of T cells	8. Immune function	8. Immediate vicinity of the central artery

Red pulps are composed of:

9. Splenic cords (cords of Billroth): Network of reticular cells, lymphocytes, macrophages, and plasma cells in reticular connective tissue	9. Screen blood and destroy irregular erythrocytes	9. Throughout red pulp of the spleen, in between the sinusoids
10. Splenic sinuses: Sinusoids lined by long, parallel endothelial cells	10. Filtration of blood and destruction of irregular erythrocytes	10. Throughout red pulp of the spleen, in between splenic cords

Additional Concepts

- **Spleen:** A unique organ that serves both the lymphoid system (providing immunologic function) and the circulatory system (filtering blood, destroying erythrocytes, undergoing hematopoiesis when induced).

- **Open circulation:** Process through which the spleen releases blood from the central artery into the splenic cord, maximizing exposure of blood cells to macrophages. Healthy erythrocytes can easily pass through the sinusoidal endothelial cells to return to circulation, whereas irregular, older cells are trapped in the cords and soon engulfed by macrophages.
- **Closed circulation:** Process through which the spleen carries blood from the central artery into the splenic sinusoids; the blood is then directly returned to circulation.

Clinical Significance

- **Splenomegaly:** An enlargement of the spleen that may occur as the spleen performs its normal function or as a result of a variety of pathologic conditions such as sarcoidosis, leukemia, etc.
- **Autosplenectomy:** Splenic tissue loss as a result of multiple infarction of the spleen. Patients with sickle cell anemia often present with autosplenectomy as the result of repeated episodes of abnormal blood cells clogging small vessels and causing infarction of the tissue downstream. Patients are more susceptible to fulminant bacterial infections.

HISTOLOGIC LOOK-A-LIKES

	Lymph Node	Thymus	Spleen
Parenchymal organization	Cortex: Lymphoid nodules in outer cortex Medulla: Medullary cords and sinuses	Cortex: Densely cellular but no lymphoid nodules Medulla: Hassall corpuscles. No cords or sinuses	White pulps: Lymphoid follicles with central arteries Red pulps: Splenic cords and sinuses
Erythrocytes	Few	Few	Abundant
Unique features	Subdivision of cortex into outer and inner cortex	Hassall corpuscles in the medulla	No cortex or medulla Lymphoid follicles with peripheral central arteries

Integumentary System | 8

INTRODUCTION

The integumentary system is composed of skin, which is comprised of the epidermis and dermis. Found within skin are numerous accessory structures such as glands, sensory structures, hair, and nails. The hypodermis lies deep to the dermis and is often composed of adipose connective tissue; though it is not a part of the skin, sensory and accessory structures of the skin may be found in this layer. Skin can be classified into thick and thin skin.

THE INTEGUMENTARY SYSTEM

THICK SKIN		
Structure	**Function**	**Location**
Epidermis		
Keratinized strati-fied squamous epithelium composed mostly of keratinocytes that are orga-nized into five layers, or strata:	Protection from friction and des-iccation	Palms and soles
1. Corneum: Keratinized, anucleate cells	1. Protection and water-proofing	Superficial
2. Lucidum: Newly keratinized, anucleate cells	2. Protection and water-proofing	
3. Granulosum: Flattening cells filled with keratohyaline granules	3. Keratin fiber organization, initiation of keratinization	Deep

(continued)

THICK SKIN (continued)		
Structure	**Function**	**Location**
Epidermis		
4. Spinosum: Mature keratinocytes	4. Keratinocyte maturation	
5. Basale: Single layer of cuboidal stem cells and melanocytes	5. Where skin stem cells and melanocytes reside	

Dermis		
Connective tissues organized into two layers:	Provide support to epidermis and connect it to hypodermis	Deep to epidermis
1. Papillary dermis: Loose connective tissue	1. Contain blood and nerve supplies to the epidermis; cushion; shock absorption	1. Superficial 20% of the dermis
2. Reticular dermis: Dense, irregular connective tissue	2. Structural support, strength and elasticity	2. Deep 80% of the dermis

Additional Concepts

- **Dermal papillae:** Finger-like papillary dermal tissue extensions increase surface area for epidermal and dermal contact. At sites that encounter high mechanical stress, dermal papillae are longer and closely packed.
- **Dermal ridges:** Longer than dermal papillae, these dermal extensions form a distinct pattern unique to each individual and are the histologic structures that cause fingerprints on the epidermal surface.

MNEMONIC

Come, Let's Get Sun-Burned!

This phrase corresponds to the layers of thick skin epidermis from superficial to deep. The layers are:

- Stratum **C**orneum
- Stratum **L**ucidum
- Stratum **G**ranulosum
- Stratum **S**pinosum
- Stratum **B**asale

THIN SKIN			
Structure		**Function**	**Location**
Epidermis			
Keratinized stratified squamous epithelium composed mostly of keratinocytes that are organized into four layers (no stratum lucidum).		Protection from friction and desiccation	All skin except for palms and soles
1. Corneum: Keratinized, anucleate cells 2. Granulosum: Flattening cells filled with keratohyaline granules 3. Spinosum: Mature keratinocytes 4. Basale: Single layer of cuboidal stem cells and melanocytes		1. Protection and water-proofing 2. Keratin fiber organization, initiation of keratinization 3. Keratinocyte maturation 4. Where skin stem cells and melanocytes reside	Superficial ↓ Deep

(continued)

THIN SKIN (continued)		
Structure	Function	Location
Dermis		
Connective tissues organized into two layers:	Provide support to epidermis and connect it to hypodermis	Deep to epidermis
1. Papillary dermis: Loose connective tissue	1. Contain blood and nerve supplies to the epidermis; cushion; shock absorption	1. Superficial 20% of the dermis
2. Reticular dermis: Dense, irregular connective tissue	2. Structural support, strength and elasticity	2. Deep 80% of the dermis

Additional Concepts

HISTOLOGIC LOOK-A-LIKES

	Thick Skin	Thin Skin
Epidermis	Five layers	Four layers (no stratum lucidum)
Accessory structures	Eccrine sweat glands, no hair	Hair, skin-associated glands

EPIDERMAL–MELANIN UNIT

A group of keratinocytes that are supplied with melanosomes from a single melanocyte. The size of the unit varies in different parts of the body.

Clinical Significance

Three types of skin cancer can arise from the epidermis:

- **Basal cell carcinoma:** Most common, but most benign of the three; arises from stratum basale
- **Squamous cell carcinoma:** Second-most common and more aggressive than basal cell carcinoma

- **Melanoma:** Arises from melanocytes of stratum basale and is the most serious form

SENSORY AND ACCESSORY STRUCTURES OF THE SKIN

SENSORY STRUCTURES			
Structure		Function	Location
Merkel cells			
Dendritic epidermal cells in the stratum basale; associated with afferent nerve fibers		Sensitive mechanoreceptors for fine touch and vibration	Stratum basale Most abundant in skin area of acute sensory perception: Fingertips, lips, clitoris, glans penis
Pacinian corpuscles			
Large spherical structures: Unmyelinated nerve ending surrounded by thick Schwann cells and capsular concentric lamellae		Receptors for deep pressure and vibration	Reticular dermis and hypodermis throughout body
Meissner corpuscles			
Small ovoid structures: Unmyelinated nerve endings surrounded by Schwann cells in spiraling layers		Receptors for low-frequency stimuli	Papillary layer of hairless skin: Lips, palms, and soles

(continued)

SENSORY STRUCTURES (continued)

Structure	Function	Location
Ruffini's corpuscles		
Fusiform structures: Thin capsule surrounding unmyelinated nerve endings suspended in fluid	Receptors for stretch and torque	Reticular dermis throughout body

ACCESSORY STRUCTURES

Structure	Function	Location
Hair		
Hair shaft: Specialized keratinized cells forming 4, 5, 6 (cuticle, cortex, and medulla) Hair root: Portion of hair inside hair follicle	Protection, sensory roles, temperature regulation	All over skin surface except palms, soles, lips, clitoris, and penis
Hair follicle		
Hair follicle: Composed of specialized epithelium supplied by dermal papilla: 1. Glassy membrane 2. External root sheath 3. Internal root sheath 4. Cuticle 5. Cortex 6. Medulla	Production and growth of hair 1. Form follicle-dermis boundary 2. Continuous with epidermis 3. Keratin production 4. Outer layer of the hair shaft 5. Form bulk of the hair 6. Core of hair	Reticular dermis and/or hypodermis Medulla is only seen in thick hairs

Structure		Function	Location
Arrector pili muscle			
Smooth muscle strips associated with hair follicles		Contract to raise hair in response to cold or sympathetic stimuli	Run between hair follicle and papillary dermis
Nail			
1. Nail plate: Specialized stratum corneum		1. Protection, support, traction	1. Tip of finger
2. Nail root: Embedded part of nail plate		2. Newly forming nail substance is added here.	2. Under the skin
3. Nail matrix: Specialized stratum basale and spinosum producing nail		3. Produce the nail and nail bed	3. Under the nail root
4. Nail bed: Specialized stratum spinosum		4. Support and protect overlying nail plate	4. Under the nail plate
5. Eponychium: Stratum corneum near nail root		5. Waterproof, fuse skin and nail plate	5. Between skin and beginning of the nail plate
6. Hyponychium: Stratum corneum under free-hanging nail		6. Waterproof barrier	6. Between free edge of the nail and the skin

(continued)

ACCESSORY STRUCTURES (continued)

Structure		Function	Location

Sebaceous glands

| Branched acinar exocrine glands composed of polygonal, vesicular cells that undergo holocrine secretion | 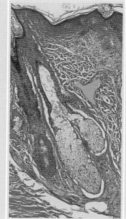 | Secrete oily and waxy secretion (sebum) with antibacterial and water-proof properties to coat the hair and skin surrounding it | Almost always associated with hair follicles Specialized sebaceous glands in eyelids: Meibomian glands |

Eccrine sweat glands

Simple coiled tubular and composed of distinct:

| 1. Secretory portion: Simple cuboidal epithelium with larger, pale-staining cells | 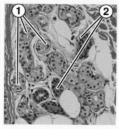 | 1. Produce watery sweat with electrolytes. Cools body temperature at evaporation | 1. All over the skin in the dermis and hypodermis except for the lips, glans penis, prepuce, clitoris, and labia minora |
| 2. Ductal portion: Stratified cuboidal epithelium with smaller, darker-staining cells | | 2. Conduct sweat directly to the surface of the skin | 2. Concentrated in palms and soles |

Structure	Function	Location
Apocrine sweat glands		
Simple coiled tubular and composed of: 1. Secretory portion: Simple cuboidal epithelium with eosinophilic cells lining large lumen 2. Ductal portion: Stratified cuboidal epithelium and drain into hair follicle	 1. Produce viscous secretion with organic compounds 2. Conduct secretions and drain into hair follicle	Dermis and hypodermis of the skin of axilla, genitalia, anus, and nipples

Additional Concepts

HISTOLOGIC LOOK-A-LIKES

	Eccrine Sweat Gland	Apocrine Sweat Gland
Morphology	• Small lumen • Pale-staining secretory cells • Numerous coiled ducts intermixed with secretory units • Ducts open directly into skin surface	• Large lumen often with secretory products • Eosinophilic secretory cells • Ducts are not commonly intermixed with secretory units • Ducts often drain into hair follicle canal
Location	All skin except for lips and portions of genitalia	Only in the skin of axilla, genitalia, anus, and around nipples

INNERVATION OF SWEAT GLANDS

Both are innervated by the autonomic nervous system:

- **Eccrine glands** are innervated by cholinergic neurons and respond to heat and stress.
- **Apocrine glands** are innervated by adrenergic neurons and respond to emotional and sensory stimuli.

Clinical Significance

- **Acne:** With increasing sebum production at puberty, sebaceous gland ducts in hair follicles may be clogged, irritated, or colonized by bacteria, causing acne lesions.
- **Body odor:** Although apocrine secretions are odorless, when bacteria on the skin surface metabolize organic contents of the secretion, odor is generated.
- **Sweat** produced by eccrine sweat glands may indicate a sign of disease.
  - **Cystic fibrosis:** Sweat is often hypertonic due to high sodium and chloride content.
  - **Uremia:** In advanced kidney failure, excess urea is released in sweat.

Digestive System | 9

INTRODUCTION

The digestive system is composed of the alimentary (gastrointestinal) canal, a long and convoluted tube that transports the ingested content from the oral cavity to the anal orifice, and a set of accessory glands that secrete lubricants, digestive enzymes, and other products to aid in the process of digestion. The alimentary canal is compartmentalized and specialized to ensure proper storage, pathogen control, and maximum absorption of nutrients.

THE DIGESTIVE SYSTEM

ORAL CAVITY		
Structure	**Function**	**Location**
Lining		
1. Lining mucosa: Nonkeratinized stratified squamous epithelium	1. Protecting the oral mucosa in areas not heavily affected by abrasion	1. Buccal membrane, soft palate, uvula, underside of the tongue, inner lips
2. Masticatory mucosa: Slightly keratinized stratified squamous epithelium	2. Protecting the oral mucosa in areas that encounter frequent friction, force, and abrasion	2. Hard palate, gingiva

(continued)

125

ORAL CAVITY (continued)

Structure	Function	Location

Lining

3. Specialized mucosa: Keratinized and nonkeratinized projections

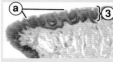

3. Providing friction to manipulate and taste food

3. Dorsum of the tongue

a. Filiform papillae: Small, numerous, keratinized projections

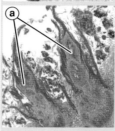

a. Providing friction, protecting from abrasion

a. Throughout dorsal surface of the tongue

b. Fungiform papillae: Mushroom-like nonkeratinized projections

b. Housing taste buds on the superior surface

b. Throughout dorsal surface of the tongue, more numerous toward the tip of the tongue

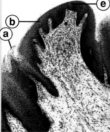

c. Foliate papillae: Ridge-like projections

c. Housing taste buds on the lateral walls

c. On posterolateral surfaces of the tongue

d. Circumvallate papillae: Large, round projections surrounded by circumferential grooves

d. Housing taste buds on the lateral walls

d. In one row, anterior to sulcus terminalis of the tongue

e. Taste buds: Pale-staining oval special sensory receptor

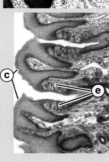

e. Relaying special sensory information to the central nervous system (CNS)

e. In fungiform, foliate, and circumvallate papillae

Structure		Function	Location
Lining			
f. Serous (Von Ebner) glands: Largely acinar exocrine glands		f. Producing watery secretion to dissolve tastants and to remove them from the folds and grooves of the tongue	f. In connective tissue underlying foliate and circumvallate papillae
Tooth			
1. Enamel: Acellular, highly mineralized, hardest substance in the body		1. Withstanding force and repeated friction to shear and tear food during mastication	1. Outermost layer of the crown
2. Dentin: Mineralized, eosinophilic layer		2. Forming the bulk and shape of the tooth, withstanding force during mastication	2. Middle layer of the tooth, both in the crown and the root
a. Dentinal tubules: Narrow channels running thickness of dentin		a. Housing odontoblast processes	a. Throughout dentin

(continued)

ORAL CAVITY (continued)		
Structure	**Function**	**Location**
Tooth		
b. Odontocyte processes: Projections of odontoblasts	b. Maintaining dentin, participating in force transfer and sensory role	b. Within dentinal tubules
c. Predentin: Much less mineralized, lighter-staining area	c. Newly secreted dentin material	c. In contact with odontoblast layer of the pulp cavity
3. Cementum: Mineralized, eosinophilic, thin, bone-like tissue layer	3. Covering the outside of the root, anchoring the tooth in the socket (alveolus) via interaction with periodontal ligament	3. Outermost surface of the root
4. Pulp cavity: Loose connective tissue with abundant neurovasculature	4. Delivering neurovascular supply to the tooth	4. Core of the tooth, both in the crown and in the root
d. Odontoblasts: Basophilic columnar cells	d. Maintaining dentin, sending out odontoblast processes	d. Immediately under dentin

Structure		Function	Location
Supporting tissues of the tooth			
5. Periodontal ligament: Dense connective tissue with abundant collagen type I fibers		5. Anchoring tooth in its socket, transferring force from tooth to the bone	5. Between the alveolar bone and cementum
6. Alveolar processes: Bone tissues that project from mandible and maxilla		6. Forming tooth sockets and securing tooth	6. Mandible and maxilla, surrounding each tooth root

SALIVARY GLANDS

Structure		Function	Location
Parotid salivary glands			
Compound branched acinar exocrine glands		Production and secretion of watery saliva	Between ramus of the mandible and styloid process of the temporal bone
1. Capsule and connective tissue septa: Dense irregular connective tissue		1. Surrounding and protecting salivary gland and dividing it into lobes and lobules	1. Outer covering and internal extensions
2. Secretory acini: Spherical secretory units, serous-secreting pyramidal to cuboidal cells		2. Producing and secreting watery fluid containing amylase	2. Throughout the gland
3. Intercalated ducts: Simple cuboidal epithelium		3. Draining each secretory acinus	3. Within the lobules of the gland

(continued)

	SALIVARY GLANDS (continued)		
Structure		**Function**	**Location**
Parotid salivary glands			
4. Striated ducts: Simple columnar epithelium, subnuclear striations	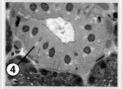	4. Draining intercalated ducts	4. Within the lobules of the gland
5. Interlobular ducts: Simple to stratified columnar epithelium		5. Draining each lobe and transferring saliva to the oral cavity	5. Within inter-lobular and interlobar septa
Submandibular salivary gland			
Compound tubuloacinar exocrine glands with more serous- than mucous-secret-ing units		Production and secretion of seromucous saliva	Submandibular triangle of the neck
1. Capsules and septa: Dense irregular con-nective tissue		1. Surrounding and protect-ing salivary gland and dividing it into lobes and lobules	1. Outer cov-ering and internal extensions
2. Secretory units		2. Production of saliva	2. Throughout the gland
a. Serous acini: Dark-staining cuboidal to pyramidal cells		a. Secretion of watery fluid con-taining amylase	
b. Mucous tubules: Clear-staining columnar cells		b. Mucous secretion	

Structure	Function	Location
Submandibular salivary gland		
c. Serous demilunes: Mucous tubules capped by serous-secreting acinar-forming hemispheres	c. Serous and mucous secretion	
3. Intercalated ducts: Simple cuboidal epithelium	3. Draining each secretory acinus	3. Within the lobules of the gland
4. Striated ducts: Simple columnar epithelium, subnuclear striations	4. Draining intercalated ducts	4. Within the lobules of the gland
5. Interlobular ducts: Simple to stratified columnar epithelium	5. Draining each lobe	5. Within interlobular and interlobar septa
Sublingual salivary glands		
Compound tubuloacinar exocrine glands with more mucous- than serous-secreting units	Production and secretion of mostly mucinous saliva	Within floor of the oral cavity
1. Capsules and septa: Dense irregular connective tissue	1. Surrounding and protecting salivary gland and dividing it into lobes and lobules	1. Outer covering and internal extensions

(continued)

SALIVARY GLANDS (continued)

Structure		Function	Location
Sublingual salivary glands			
2. Mostly mucous tubules with some serous demilunes	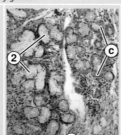	2. Production of saliva, mostly mucus with a little serous content	2. Throughout the gland
3. Intercalated ducts: Simple cuboidal epithelium		3. Draining each secretory acinus	3. Within the lobules of the gland
4. Striated ducts: Simple cuboidal to columnar epithelium, subnuclear striations		4. Draining intercalated ducts	4. Within the lobules of the gland
5. Interlobular ducts: Simple to stratified columnar epithelium		5. Draining each lobe	5. Within interlobular and interlobar septa

GENERAL HISTOLOGY OF THE GASTROINTESTINAL TRACT*

Structure		Function	Location
Layers			
1. Mucosa: Composed of three layers	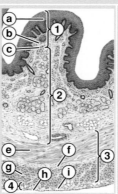	1. Lining and protecting the lumen, absorption and secretion	1. Innermost layer

Structure	Function	Location
Layers		
a. Epithelium: Varies depending on location between nonkeratinized stratified squamous epithelium to simple columnar epithelium	a. Lining and protecting the mucosa, secretion and absorption	a. In contact with lumen
b. Lamina propria: Loose connective tissue to diffuse lymphoid tissue	b. Supporting the epithelium, providing immune function	b. Deep to epithelium
c. Muscularis mucosa: Thin strip of smooth muscle tissue	c. Providing movements of the mucosa independent of outer layers, aiding in gland secretion	c. Outermost layer of the mucosa
2. Submucosa: Mostly dense irregular connective tissue	2. Providing structural support	2. Between mucosa and muscularis propria
d. Submucosal (Meissner) plexus: Palestaining, oval parasympathetic ganglia	d. Delivery of parasympathetic innervations	d. Scattered throughout submucosa

(continued)

GENERAL HISTOLOGY OF THE GASTROINTESTINAL TRACT* (continued)

Structure	Function	Location
Layers		
3. Muscularis propria (externa): Thicker smooth muscle layers	3. Producing peristaltic movements to conduct chyme through the digestive tract	3. Between sub-mucosa and serosa
e. Circular layer: Circumfer-ential orientation	e. Sequential constric-tion of gastroin-testinal (GI) tract	e. Inner layer of muscularis propria
f. Myenteric (Auerbach) plexus: Pale-staining, oval parasympa-thetic gan-glia	f. Delivery of para-sympa-thetic innerva-tions	f. Between circular and lon-gitudinal layers of muscularis propria
g. Longitudi-nal layer: Runs paral-lel to long axis of the digestive tract • Oblique layer in the stomach, runs obliquely	g. Wave-like contrac-tion through the length of GI tract • Churn-ing of the food	g. Outer layer of muscularis propria
4. Serosa: Connective tissue	4. Covering, delivering neurovas-cular sup-port to the outside of the GI tract	4. Outer layer to muscularis propria in most intra-peritoneal portions of GI tract

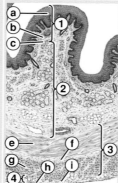

Structure	Function	Location
Layers		
h. Mesothelium: Simple squamous epithelium, visceral layer of peritoneum	h. Producing serous fluid	h. Outermost layer of the GI tract
i. Subserosa: Loose to adipose connective tissue	i. Supporting, insulating GI tract	i. Between mesothelium and muscularis propria
• Adventitia: Connective tissue without mesothelium		• Outermost layer of mediastinal esophagus, portions of duodenum and ascending and descending colons and rectum

*Also known as the alimentary canal, GI or digestive tract.

Additional Concepts

- **Mucosa:** May be considered as a skin equivalent inside the body. It covers all areas within the body that come in contact with the outside environment and foreign molecules. Much like the skin, which has an epithelium (epidermis), a connective tissue layer (dermis), and accessory glands and structures (sweat glands, hair), mucosa too has sublayers (epithelium, lamina propria, muscularis mucosa) and associated glands. Similar to skin, mucosa plays a critical role in host defense by physically preventing pathogens from entering the body and immunologically responding to antigens. The epithelium of the GI tract is protective, nonkeratinized stratified squamous at the ends and absorptive and secretory simple columnar epithelium in between.

ESOPHAGUS

Structure		Function	Location
Layers			
Long, muscular, flexible tube with collapsed lumen when not in use		Conducting ingested bolus from oral cavity to stomach, preventing reflux when not in use	Extending from pharynx to stomach, behind trachea, most of the segment in mediastinum, short terminal segment in peritoneum
1. Mucosa: Thrown into longitudinal folds with collapsed lumen		1. Protecting, distending and collapsing the lumen as bolus passes	1. Luminal layer
a. Epithelium: Nonkeratinized stratified squamous epithelium		a. Protecting, withstanding friction during swallowing	a. In contact with lumen
b. Lamina propria: Loose connective tissue		b. Nutritional, immunologic support for epithelium	b. Deep to epithelium
c. Muscularis mucosa: Smooth muscle tissue		c. Contributing to mucosal folding	c. Outermost mucosal layer
2. Submucosa: Dense irregular connective tissue		2. Structural support, delivery of neurovasculature to the esophageal wall	2. Between muscularis mucosa and propria
d. Esophageal glands: Compound tubuloacinar exocrine glands		d. Secreting mucus, lubricating the lumen	d. Scattered throughout submucosa, increase in number closer to stomach

Structure		Function	Location
Layers			
3. Muscularis propria		3. Peristaltic contraction during swallowing	3. Between submucosa and adventitia
e. Skeletal muscles			e. Upper one-third of esophagus
f. Skeletal and smooth muscles			f. Middle one-third of esophagus
g. Smooth muscles			g. Lower one-third of esophagus
4. Adventitia or serosa: Connective tissue		4. Anchoring, stabilizing, supporting esophagus	4. Outermost layer
Gastroesophageal junction			
1. Epithelium: Abrupt transition		1. Lining and protecting mucosa	1. Innermost mucosal layer at the junction between esophagus and stomach
a. Nonkeratinized stratified squamous epithelium		a. Reduction of friction	a. Esophagus
b. Simple columnar epithelium		b. Protection from acid	b. Stomach cardia
2. Lamina propria: Abundant mucous glands in the stomach		2. Coating the epithelium with mucus to provide protection from acid	2. Lamina propria of stomach

(continued)

ESOPHAGUS (continued)		
Structure	**Function**	**Location**
Gastroesophageal junction		
3. Muscularis mucosa is thickened.	3. Providing limited sphincter-like function, limiting reflux of gastric content	3. At the junction of esophagus and stomach

Clinical Significance

- **Gastroesophageal reflux disease (GERD):** Inflammation of esophageal mucosa as the result of prolonged, repeated exposure of esophageal mucosa to the gastric acid causing symptoms such as heartburn, regurgitation, and dysphagia. A subset of GERD patients may progress and develop Barrett esophagus, characterized by the erosion of esophageal mucosa and metaplastic simple columnar epithelium formation in the lower esophagus.

STOMACH		
Structure	**Function**	**Location**
Macroscopic features		
Dilated portion of the GI tract	Temporary storage of ingested food, mixing it with stomach juice; disinfecting; initiating digestion	Left quadrant of the abdomen
1. Cardia: Ring-like region surrounding gastrointestinal junction	1. Receiving bolus from esophagus, limited prevention of reflux	1. Area surrounding the esophageal orifice
2. Fundus: Dome-shaped superior outpocketing	2. Accommodating large volume of food and drinks	2. Left superior portion of the stomach, abutting diaphragm

Structure		Function	Location
Macroscopic features			
3. Body: Majority of the stomach		3. Temporary storage, churning, mixing of food with stomach secretions	3. Majority of the midportion of the stomach
4. Pylorus: Funnel-like distal end of the stomach		4. Controlled release of chyme into duodenum, preventing reflux	4. Distal, inferior-most portion of the stomach
5. Rugae: Longitudinal mucosal folds		5. Allowing stomach to expand	5. Mostly in the body
6. Villi: Numerous mucosal projections into the lumen that give the mucosa a velvety appearance		6. Increasing surface area	6. Throughout stomach mucosa
7. Gastric pits: Hole-like depressions in between villi that are ductal openings of stomach glands		7. Releasing stomach gland secretions into the lumen	7. Throughout stomach mucosa
Cardia and pyloric histology			
1. Villi: Short mucosal projections		1. Increasing surface area	1. Throughout stomach mucosa
a. Epithelium: Simple columnar, mostly goblet cells		a. Forming a protective lining	a. Innermost layer

(continued)

STOMACH (continued)		
Structure	**Function**	**Location**

Cardia and pyloric histology

2. Lamina propria: Diffuse lymphoid tissue with occasional lymphoid follicles	2. Providing immune response to pathogens	2. Deep to epithelium
b. Glands: Branched tubular mucous-secreting exocrine glands	b. Secreting mucus to coat and protect the epithelium and contribute to gastric juice	b. Within lamina propria

Fundus and body histology

1. Villi: Slightly longer, finger-like projections lined with simple columnar goblet cells	1. Increasing surface area	1. Throughout mucosa
2. Glands: Branched tubular exocrine glands	2. Producing majority of the stomach juice	2. Lamina propria
a. Parietal cells: Eosinophilic, polygonal cells with central spherical nuclei	a. Hydrochloric acid (HCl) production, intrinsic factor secretion	a. Mid- to luminal regions of the glands
b. Chief cells: Smaller basophilic cells with heterochromatic small nuclei	b. Pepsinogen production	b. Deeper, basal regions of the glands

Clinical Significance

- **Gastric ulcer:** A gastric mucosal defect that extends through the muscularis mucosa when the protective mechanisms of the mucosa are altered by *Helicobacter pylori* infection or prolonged and repeated exposure to alcohol, bile salts, and acid.
- **Intrinsic factor:** Critical for absorption of vitamin B_{12} in the small intestine. A decrease in intrinsic factor and insufficient vitamin B_{12}, which plays an important role in erythropoiesis, may result in development of pernicious anemia.

SMALL INTESTINE		
Structure	**Function**	**Location**
Macroscopic features		
Long, convoluted tube of uniform diameter divided into three segments with nondistinct border but distinct histologic difference: Duodenum, jejunum, and ileum	Main site of digestion, absorption, and secretion	Largely in the middle of the abdominal cavity
1. Plicae circulares: Large, horizontal projections a. Submucosal core	1. Loosely compartmentalizing small intestine, increasing surface area	1. Throughout small intestine, most prominent and numerous in jejunum
2. Villi: Numerous long, fingerlike mucosal projections into the lumen that give the mucosa a velvety appearance b. Lamina propria core	2. Increasing surface area for absorption and secretion	2. Throughout small intestinal mucosa

SMALL INTESTINE (continued)

Structure	Function	Location

Macroscopic features

3. Crypts of Lieberkühn: Deep depressions in between villi that are ductal openings of intestinal glands 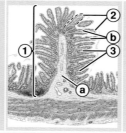	3. Releasing intestinal gland secretions into the lumen	3. Throughout small intestinal mucosa

Cells of the small intestine

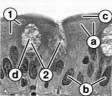

1. Enterocytes: Columnar cells
  a. Eosinophilic cytoplasm
  b. Basal nuclei
  c. Microvilli
	1. Absorption	1. Throughout small intestine, most abundant in jejunum

2. Goblet cells: Pale-staining columnar cells d. Apical mucous-filled vesicles	2. Mucous secretion	2. Increase in number toward distal intestine

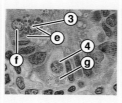

3. Paneth cells: Columnar cells
  e. Abundant supranuclear eosinophilic granules in cytoplasm
  f. Basal nuclei
	3. Antibacterial function, phagocytosis of bacteria, regulating normal flora	3. Base of the intestinal glands

4. Enteroendocrine cells: Columnar cells g. Infranuclear eosinophilic granules	4. Releasing hormones to regulate digestion	4. Base of the intestinal glands

Structure		Function	Location
Cells of the small intestine			
5. M cells: Columnar cells, no microvilli		5. Antigen transport, engulfing microorganisms, immune function	5. In lining epithelium overlying Peyer patches
Duodenum			
First, short segment of small intestine		Neutralizing acidic chime, mixing it with pancreatic secretions	Retroperitoneal position behind the liver and loops of distal small intestine
1. Plicae circulares: Moderate amount		1. Limited compartmentalization of duodenum	1. Throughout duodenum
2. Villi: Leaf-like, midlength mucosal projections		2. Increasing surface area	2. Throughout duodenal mucosa
3. Epithelium: Simple columnar epithelium		3. Protection, limited amount of absorption	3. Innermost mucosal layer in contact with duodenal content
4. Brunner glands: Branched tubuloacinar glands		4. Secretion of alkaline glycoproteins, bicarbonate ions, mucus, and zymogens	4. Duodenal submucosa

(continued)

SMALL INTESTINE (continued)

Structure	Function	Location

Jejunum

Middle, longest portion of the small intestine	Majority of absorption	Within the peritoneum
1. Plicae circulares: Prominent and numerous	1. Limited compartmentalization of jejunum	1. Throughout jejunum
2. Villi: Long, finger-like mucosal projections	2. Increasing surface area	2. Throughout jejunal mucosa
3. Epithelium: Simple columnar with mostly enterocytes	3. Absorption of nutrients	3. Innermost mucosal layer in contact with jejunal content
4. Intestinal glands: Simple to branched tubular, relatively uniform in size and shape	4. Production of seromucous secretions	4. Lamina propria

Ileum

Last segment of small intestine	Absorbing vitamin B_{12}, bile salts, other nutrients remaining in chyme	Lower portion of the peritoneum
1. Plicae circulares: Decrease in number and height toward distal portion	1. Limited compartmentalization of ileum	1. Throughout ileum
2. Villi: Long, finger-like mucosal projections	2. Increasing surface area	2. Throughout ileal mucosa

Structure	Function	Location
Ileum		
3. Epithelium: Simple columnar with increasing goblet cells	3. Absorption of nutrients, mucous secretion	3. Innermost mucosal layer in contact with ileal content
4. Intestinal glands: Simple to branched tubular, relatively uniform size and shape	4. Seromucous secretion	4. Lamina propria, may extend into submucosa
5. Peyer patches: Large lymphoid follicles with or without germinal centers	5. Immune surveillance and response to encountered antigens	5. In lining epithelium over Peyer patches
a. M cells on the overlying epithelium	a. Antigen transport, engulfing microorganisms, immune function	

Additional Concepts

Structures that increase the surface area in small intestine:

- **Plicae circulares:** Macroscopic, submucosal projections into the lumen. The submucosal tissue forms the core of the plicae and is covered by the mucosa, containing villi.
- **Villi:** Microscopic mucosal projections into the lumen. Lamina propria forms the core of the villous projections.
- **Microvilli:** Microscopic, apical cellular projections into the lumen, forming the brush border and responsible for increasing the surface area of the small intestine the most.

LARGE INTESTINE (COLON)

Structure	Function	Location
Macroscopic features		
Larger tube of varying diameters, six segments (cecum; ascending, transverse, descending, sigmoid colons; rectum), and an appendix. The histology of the six segments are almost identical.	Water and vitamin absorption, compaction and storage of fecal matter	Both peritoneal (cecum, appendix, transverse colon, and sigmoid colon) and retroperitoneal (ascending and descending colons and rectum)
1. Teniae coli: Three longitudinal strips of smooth muscles	1. Aiding in peristalsis, forming haustra	1. Throughout the length of large intestine except for appendix and rectum
2. Haustra: Small saccules of large intestine	2. Limited compartmentalization of the colon, moving fecal matter in a segmental fashion	2. Throughout the length of large intestine except for appendix and rectum
3. Epiploic appendages: Saccules of fat tissue attached to outer surface	3. No obvious function	3. Outside of colon
4. No plicae circulares	4. Haustra rather than plicae circulares segment the colon	
5. Little to no villi	5. Reduction in surface area in contact with fecal matter	

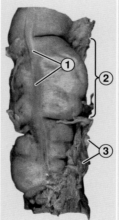

Structure		Function	Location
Microscopic features			
1. Mucosa: Relatively thin		1. Absorption, protection, lubrication	1. Inner layer of colonic wall
a. Epithelium: Simple columnar		a. Lining the lumen, absorption of mostly water	a. Innermost mucosal layer, in contact with lumen
b. Lamina propria: Diffuse lymphoid tissue and lymphoid follicles		b. Immunologic surveillance, response to antigens	b. Deep to epithelium
c. Glands: Simple tubular glands		c. Production of mucus	c. Within lamina propria
d. Muscularis mucosa: Thin strip of smooth muscle layer		d. Isolated movements of mucosa	d. Outermost mucosal layer
2. Submucosa: Dense irregular connective tissue		2. Structural support, delivery of neurovasculature	2. Between muscularis mucosa and propria
3. Muscularis propria		3. Peristaltic movements	3. Between submucosa and serosa
e. Circular layer: Smooth muscle tissue		e. Constriction of compartments	
f. Longitudinal layer: Smooth muscle tissue, thickened bands (teniae coli)		f. Longitudinal contraction, maintaining haustra	

(continued)

LARGE INTESTINE (COLON) (continued)

Structure	Function	Location

Microscopic features

4. Serosa or adventitia: Connective tissue with or without mesothelium	4. Protection, insulation, delivery of neurovasculature	4. Outermost layer

Appendix

Similar histology as the rest of the large intestine except for:	Largely immunologic surveillance and immune response	Extending out from inferior portion of cecum, position with the peritoneum varies
1. Uniform, longitudinal layer instead of teniae coli	1. Unclear	1. Outer layer of muscularis propria
2. Large number of lymphoid nodules with or without germinal center	2. Phagocytosis, antibody production, lymphocyte proliferation and differentiation	2. Lamina propria and submucosa

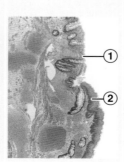

Anorectal junction

Site of mucosal transition	Lining and protecting the mucosa at the site of transition	Junction between terminal segment of rectum and anal column
1. Simple columnar, colonic epithelium	1. Lining, lubricating lumen	

Structure	Function	Location
Anorectal junction		
2. Nonkeratinized stratified squamous epithelium, eventually transitioning to keratinized stratified squamous of the perianal skin	2. Protecting from abrasion and friction	

Clinical Significance

- **Appendicitis:** Inflammation of the appendix often as the result of luminal obstruction from fecaliths, lymphoid hyperplasia, or infection. Common symptoms of an acute event include anorexia, pain in the right upper quadrant, nausea, and vomiting. Appendectomy is the only curative treatment.
- **Diverticulitis:** Inflammation of diverticula and small herniations of the intestinal wall. Diverticula commonly occur in the large intestine in areas of wall weakness, such as entry/exit points for neurovasculature through the wall and areas in between teniae coli. In the event of obstruction of the diverticular lumen, acute inflammation, necrosis, and even perforation of intestinal wall may result.
- **Colonic polyps:** Slow-growing benign tumors of the colonic mucosa that may become malignant with increasing size, number, and occurrence. Certain histologic features of the polyps such as villous and secretory morphology are associated with high morbidity and mortality; hence, regular screening of the colon for the presence of polyps is an important preventative medical practice in the Western world.

HISTOLOGIC LOOK-A-LIKES

Duodenum	Jejunum	Ileum	Colon
Mucosa			
Leaf-like villi	Prominent, numerous, and high plicae circulares; long and finger-like villi	Shorter, finger-like villi; abundant goblet cells in lining and glandular epithelia; Peyer patches present	Little to no villi, abundant goblet cells in lining and glandular epithelia, simple tubular glands, no Paneth cells
Submucosa			
Brunner glands are present	No glands	Peyer patches may extend into submucosa, no glands	No glands
Muscularis propria			
Two uniform layers	Two uniform layers	Two uniform layers	Outer longitudinal layer forms three bands (teniae coli) rather than a uniform layer

LIVER		
Structure	**Function**	**Location**
Macroscopic features		
Large, brown, red organ. Four lobes: 1. Right lobe 2. Left lobe 3. Quadrate lobe 4. Caudate lobe	Over 200 functions. Functions related to digestive system include filtration of blood, detoxification, gluconeogenesis, and bile production.	Right upper quadrant of peritoneum, superior margin in contact with diaphragm
Hepatic lobule		
Hexagonal structural unit of the liver	Structural division of the liver	Throughout liver
1. Central vein: Endothelium	1. Draining blood from sinusoids	1. Center of each lobule

Structure		Function	Location
Hepatic lobule			
2. Hepatic portal triad: Three channels embedded in connective tissue		2. Delivering blood to and draining bile from the lobule	2. Each corner of the hexagonal lobule
a. Hepatic arteriole: Small lumen, one to two smooth muscles		a. Delivering oxygenated blood	
b. Hepatic venule: Largest of the three channels, one to two smooth muscles		b. Delivering oxygen-poor blood from hepatic portal system	
c. Bile duct: Simple cuboidal epithelium		c. Draining bile from canaliculi	

(continued)

LIVER (continued)

Structure	Function	Location

Microscopic features

3. Hepatocytes: Large, polygonal cells that form a cord or plate of hepatic lobule

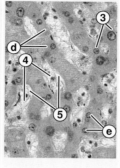

3. Modification, storage of nutrients, detoxification of blood, gluconeogenesis, production and secretion of bile

3. Throughout liver in cords or plates between sinusoids

   d. Cytoplasm: Large, eosinophilic cytoplasm with lipid or glycogen granules

   d. Metabolism

   d. Major component of hepatocytes

   e. Nuclei: Large, euchromatic, spherical, distinct nucleoli

   e. Maintenance of cellular structure and function

   e. Central to slightly eccentric area of the cell

   f. Canaliculi: Small, narrow channels between neighboring hepatocytes, formed by tight junctions

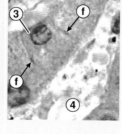

   f. Draining bile and conducting it to bile ducts

   f. In between hepatocytes

4. Sinusoids: Endothelium with large gaps between cells and incomplete basement membrane

4. Channeling blood from hepatic portal vein and hepatic artery toward central vein; filtering, detoxifying, and regulating the amount of nutrient

4. In between the plates or cords of hepatocytes

Structure	Function	Location
Microscopic features		
g. Kupffer cells: Resident macrophages of the liver, stellate to ovoid	g. Phagocytosis of pathogens, debris, damaged erythrocytes	g. Within the sinusoidal space
5. Perisinusoidal space: Narrow space between sinusoidal endothelial cell and hepatocytes	5. Retention of blood and other molecules for processing	5. Between hepatocytes and endothelium of sinusoids

Additional Concepts
Three ways to divide the liver (FIG. 9-1):

- **Hepatic lobules:** Hexagonal, morphologic division with the central vein in the center and approximately six hepatic portal triads in each corner of the hexagon. Easily recognizable, structural division in which blood travels from each corner of the hexagon and drains into the central vein and bile travels from the vicinity of the central vein toward bile ducts in the periphery.
- **Portal lobule:** Triangular division with a single hepatic portal triad in the center and three central veins in each corner. Bile pathway–centered view in which bile from the central vein in the center of the portal lobule is drained toward each side of the abutting hepatic portal triad.
- **Hepatic acinus:** Two adjacent triangular wedges of two hepatic lobules with the linear hepatic portal triad track in the middle and two central veins at each apex of each triangle. Blood pathway–centered view in which oxygenated and nutrient-rich blood from the hepatic portal tract drains toward the opposite poles, further dividing the hepatic tissue into three pairs of zones.

Clinical Significance
- **Liver cirrhosis:** Diffuse fibrosis (scarring) of the liver resulting from diverse causes such as hepatitis C infection and repeated and

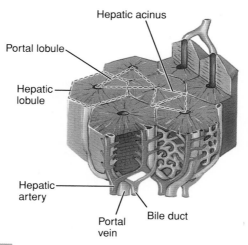

Hepatic acinus

Portal lobule

Hepatic lobule

Hepatic artery

Portal vein

Bile duct

Figure 9-1. Hepatic divisions. (From Gartner LP, Hiatt JL. *Color Atlas of Histology*. 5th ed. Baltimore: Lippincott Williams & Wilkins, 2009:326.)

prolonged exposure to noxious and carcinogenic chemicals. Due to the liver's diverse and many critical roles in the body, severe cases of liver cirrhosis are associated with high morbidity and mortality. Complications of liver cirrhosis include portal hypertension, ascites, hepatorenal syndrome, and hepatic encephalopathy.

- **Complications of hepatic portal hypertension:** Increased hepatic portal pressure causes venous blood returning from the GI tract to take an alternate route back to the systemic circulation. Three major anastomotic sites between the portal and systemic vasculature are hence affected, resulting in:
  - **Esophageal varices:** Varicose vein of the esophagus. Due to nonkeratinized lining and frequent abrasion by the passing bolus, esophageal varices may tear easily and cause massive upper gastrointestinal hemorrhage.
  - **Caput medusae:** Varicose paraumbilical veins form a radiating pattern from the umbilicus.
  - **Rectal hemorrhoids:** Varicose veins in rectal mucosa near the anorectal junction.

GALL BLADDER

Structure		Function	Location
Layers			
Bile-stained (green), oval, blind pouch		Storage, concentration, regulation of bile	Inferior surface of the liver
1. Mucosa: Multiple folds project into the lumen.		1. Lining and protecting mucosa	1. Inner layer of gall bladder
a. Epithelium: Simple columnar epithelium		a. Lining mucosa, limited amount of absorption	a. Innermost layer in contact with bile in lumen
b. Lamina propria: Loose connective tissue, little to no glands		b. Supporting epithelium, delivery of neurovasculature	b. Deep to epithelium
2. Muscularis externa: Smooth muscles		2. Contraction and injection of bile into duodenum	2. Deep to lamina propria
3. Serosa and adventitia: Connective tissue with or without mesothelium		3. Covering, insulating, protecting gall bladder	3. Outermost layer of gall bladder
• No muscularis mucosa or submucosa			

PANCREAS			
Structure		**Function**	**Location**
Macroscopic features			
Elongated fleshy organ		Production and secretion of digestive enzymes into duodenum, secretion of digestive hormones into bloodstream	Retroperitoneal position medial to the lesser curvature of duodenum
1. Head: Dilated right end of pancreas		1–3. Secretion of digestive enzymes and hormones	1. In contact with and medial to the duodenal curvature
a. Uncinate process: Bulbous inferior portion of the head			a. Inferior-posterior extension of the head
2. Body: Long midportion of the gland			2. Extend from the head toward the spleen
3. Tail: Tapered end of pancreas			3. Left, distal end close to spleen
4. Pancreatic duct: Runs the length of the gland and drains into the lumen of the duodenum		4. Draining exocrine glands of pancreas and delivering secretions to duodenum	4. Runs in the center throughout length of the pancreas, makes a sharp downward angle near the head

Structure		Function	Location
Macroscopic features			
5. Accessory pancreatic duct: Short and straight continuation of the main pancreatic duct that opens proximal to the main pancreatic duct		5. Present in some portion of population, draining portions of exocrine pancreas	5. Straight continuation of the main pancreatic duct in the head
6. Hepatopancreatic sphincter (of Oddi)		6. Regulating flow of bile and pancreatic secretions into the duodenum, preventing reflux	6. Within duodenal wall
Microscopic features			
1. Exocrine glandular unit		1. Secreting digestive proenzymes	1. Throughout pancreas
a. Secretory acini: Cuboidal to pyramidal cells with granular cytoplasm and spherical nuclei, arranged in spherical units		a. Secreting peptidases, amylases, lipases, and nucleolytic enzymes	a. Throughout pancreas at distal ends of intercalated ducts
b. Intercalated duct: Pale-staining simple cuboidal epithelium		b. Draining exocrine acini	b. Immediately in contact with secretory acini

(continued)

PANCREAS (continued)		
Structure	Function	Location
Microscopic features		
c. Centroac- inar cells: Interca- lated duct cells within acini	c. Protruding into and draining acini	c. Within entryway into secre- tory acini
• No stri- ated ducts		
2. Pancreatic islets (of Langerhans): Pale-staining endocrine units	2. Producing and releasing hormones into blood vessels	2. Throughout pancreas
d. Alpha cells: Pale stain- ing	d. Secreting glucagon	d. Peripheral portion of the islet
e. Beta cells: More eosino- philic staining	e. Secreting insulin	e. Central portion of the islet
f. Delta cells are indis- tinct.	f. Secreting soma- tostatin	f. Peripheral regions

Clinical Significance

- **Diabetes mellitus:** A disease of glucose metabolism resulting in a variety of complications
  - **Type I:** Results from the lack of insulin production by the pan- creatic islets due to autoimmune destruction of the beta cells. Though type I diabetes mellitus can occur at any age, it is most commonly diagnosed in juveniles. Type I diabetes mellitus is not associated with obesity; patients are exogenous insulin dependent, and without insulin treatment, diabetic ketoacidosis ensues, which may progress to coma and death.
  - **Type II:** Results from insufficient insulin secretion by the beta cells in pancreatic islets or cellular resistance to insulin that causes hyperglycemia. Type II diabetes mellitus is commonly

associated with obesity and complications include diabetic reti-
nopathy, nephropathy, and neuropathy.

MNEMONIC

The relationship between pancreatic islet cells and their secretions
can be remembered based on alphabetical order. A comes before B,
and G comes before I. Therefore,

Alpha cells secrete **G**lucagon

Beta cells secrete **I**nsulin

Respiratory System | 10

INTRODUCTION

The respiratory system is composed of the conducting portion, a series of passageways that filter, condition, and deliver the air to the gas exchange surface, and the respiratory portion, the lung tissues in which actual gas exchange takes place. Lungs are highly vascular with abundant continuous capillaries in close contact with alveolar epithelium. This allows rapid exchange of oxygen and carbon dioxide between air in the alveolar space and blood in the capillary. The respiratory system also plays a role in olfaction, speech, minor hormone production, and immune response to antigens present in the inhaled air. Most of the conducting portion is lined by ciliated pseudostratified columnar epithelium, also known as the respiratory epithelium.

CONDUCTING PORTION

UPPER RESPIRATORY TRACT		
Structure	**Function**	**Location**
Nasal cavity		
1. Nasal vestibule	1. Conduit between the nasal cavity and the external environment	1. Just inside nostrils
a. Stratified squamous epithelium	a. Protection	a. Mucosal lining
b. Vibrissae	b. Trap dust and particulate matter from inhaled air	b. Throughout mucosa

(continued)

UPPER RESPIRATORY TRACT (continued)

Structure		Function	Location
Nasal cavity			
c. Sebaceous glands		c. Aid in trapping particulate matter	c. Throughout mucosa
2. Respiratory region (nasal mucosa)		2. Condition inhaled air	2. Inferior two-thirds of the nasal cavities
d. Ciliated pseudostratified columnar epithelium		d. Trap particulate matter and propel it toward nasopharynx	d. Mucosal lining
e. Rich vascular network		e. Warm the air	e. Lamina propria
f. Seromucous glands		f. Secretion aids in filtering and moistening the air.	f. Lamina propria
3. Olfactory region (olfactory mucosa)		3. Olfaction	3. Superior portion of the nasal cavity
g. Olfactory epithelium (specialized ciliated pseudostratified columnar epithelium with bipolar receptor neurons)		g. Receive and relay olfactory signals	g. Mucosal lining
h. Olfactory glands (Bowman glands)		h. Secretions trap and dissolve odoriferous particles.	h. Lamina propria
i. Axon bundles		i. Pass through cribriform plate of the ethmoid to form olfactory nerve	i. Lamina propria

Structure	Function	Location
Larynx		
Tubular structure	Conduct air between oropharynx and trachea	Anterior neck, inferior to oropharynx, superior to trachea
1. Irregular hyaline cartilage plates	1. Structural support, protection	1. Laryngeal wall
2. Epiglottis: Elastic cartilage	2. Strong yet flexible support, prevent food particles from entering the trachea	2. Entrance of the laryngeal inlet
3. Mucosal lining	3. Line the lumen	3. Lumen of the larynx
a. Respiratory epithelium	a. Trap particulate matter, propel mucus toward oropharynx	a. Most of the luminal surface
b. Nonkeratinized stratified squamous epithelium	b. Protection from friction and force	b. Mucosal linings of the true vocal cords, lingual surface and tip of epiglottis
c. Lamina propria	c. Support epithelia	c. Deep to covering epithelium
d. Glands	d. Produce seromucous secretion	d. Within lamina propria
4. False vocal cords (ventricular folds)	4. Resonance production	4. Superior to true vocal cords

(continued)

UPPER RESPIRATORY TRACT (continued)		
Structure	Function	Location
Larynx		
5. True vocal cords	5. Sound production	5. Inferior to false vocal cords
e. Vocalis muscles: Skeletal muscle tissue	e. Contract to produce various pitches	e. Core of the cord

Clinical Significance

- **Anosmia:** Loss of sense of smell that may occur when olfactory axon bundles are severed permanently. Because the axon bundles passing through cribriform plates are fragile, anosmia is not uncommon in patients with traumatic head injury.
- **Nose bleed:** Highly vascular nasal mucosa is lined by delicate respiratory epithelium rather than more protective stratified squamous epithelium; hence, bleeding from this region occurs relatively easily with dryness or varying degrees of trauma.
- **Nasal congestion:** Inflammation of the nasal mucosa as the result of allergic reaction or viral infection can restrict air conduction and cause difficulty breathing.
- **Laryngitis:** Inflammation of the laryngeal mucosa as the result of infection causes difficulty breathing and swallowing, hoarseness, and even loss of voice.
- **Age-related changes in epiglottis:** With advancing age, elastic cartilage is reduced or replaced by adipose tissue. Decreased elasticity and resulting stiffness of the epiglottis increase risk of food or liquid aspiration.

LOWER RESPIRATORY TRACT		
Structure	Function	Location
Trachea		
Long, flexible, tubular airway:	Conduct air from larynx to primary bronchi	Inferior to larynx, anterior to esophagus
1. C-shaped cartilage rings	1. Keep the lumen open	1. Throughout the length of trachea at regular intervals

Structure		Function	Location
Trachea			
2. Trachealis: Longitudinal smooth muscles		2. Narrow the lumen	2. Between the posterior opening of the C-shaped cartilage
Four layers of the wall			
3. Mucosa		3. Line the tracheal lumen	3. Luminal surface
a. Respiratory epithelium		a. Condition inhaled air, capture particles and propel them toward oropharynx	a. Mucosal surface
b. Lamina propria: Connective tissue		b. Support respiratory epithelium	b. Deep to epithelium
4. Submucosa: Loose to dense connective tissue		4. Carry bigger vessels, house bronchus-associated lymphoid tissue (BALT)	4. Deep to mucosa
c. Seromucous glands		c. Produce seromucous secretion	c. Throughout submucosa
5. Cartilage layer: Hyaline cartilage		5. Structural framework, keep the lumen open	5. Core of the tracheal wall
6. Adventitia: Connective tissue		6. Secure trachea to surrounding structures, carry bigger vessels and nerves	6. Outermost layer of the tracheal wall

(continued)

LOWER RESPIRATORY TRACT (continued)

Structure	Function	Location
Bronchi		
Series of airway branches of progressively decreasing size	Conduct air	Conducting airway branches distal to trachea
1. Mucosa	1. Line the lumen	1. Luminal surface
a. Respiratory epithelium	a. Condition inhaled air, capture particles and propel them upward	a. Mucosal surface
b. Lamina propria	b. Support respiratory epithelium	b. Deep to epithelium
2. Smooth muscle layer	2. Regulate diameter of the airway	2. Deep to mucosa
3. Submucosa: Loose connective tissue	3. Support and delivery of vessels	3. Deep to smooth muscle layer
4. Cartilage layer: Hyaline cartilage ranging from complete rings in primary bronchi to small plates or bars in terminal bronchi	4. Structural framework and support	4. Between smooth muscle layer and adventitia
5. Adventitia: Loose to dense connective tissue	5. Blend with adjacent structures	5. Outermost layer

Structure		Function	Location
Bronchioles			
Series of smaller branches from bronchi		Conduct air	Conducting branches distal to bronchi
1. Luminal epithelium		1. Line the lumen	1. Luminal surface
a. Respiratory epithelium	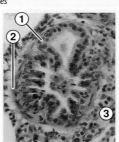	a. Condition inhaled air, capture particles and propel them upward	a. Larger bronchioles
b. Ciliated simple columnar epithelium		b. Support respiratory epithelium	b. Smaller bronchioles
c. Clara cells: Nonciliated cuboidal cells with dome-like apical projections		c. Secrete surface-active agents and antimicrobial products	c. Throughout bronchiolar epithelium, increase in number in distal bronchioles
2. Smooth muscle layer		2. Regulate diameter of the airway	2. Middle layer
3. Adventitia		3. Blend with adjacent structures	3. Outermost layer
Terminal bronchioles			
Distal-most and smallest bronchioles		Conduct air	Distal-most segment of the conduction portions
1. Simple cuboidal epithelium		1. Condition inhaled air, capture particles and propel them upward	1. Luminal surface

(continued)

LOWER RESPIRATORY TRACT (continued)		
Structure	Function	Location
Terminal bronchioles		
a. Clara cells: Nonciliated cuboidal cells with dome-like apical projections	a. Secrete surface-active agents and anti-microbial products	a. Epithelium
2. Smooth muscle layer	2. Regulate diameter of the airway	2. Middle layer
3. Adventitia	3. Blend with adjacent structures	3. Outermost layer

Clinical Significance

- **Asthma and chronic obstructive pulmonary disease (COPD)** are associated with spasms of bronchial smooth muscles. Inhalant bronchodilator medications are designed to relax smooth muscles.

HISTOLOGIC LOOK-A-LIKES

	Trachea	Bronchi	Bronchioles
Epithelium	Ciliated pseudostratified columnar epithelium	Ciliated pseudostratified columnar epithelium	Varies; ciliated pseudostratified columnar epithelium, ciliated simple columnar, and ciliated simple cuboidal epithelium depending on the size of the branch
Cartilage	C-shaped rings with trachealis muscles closing the opening of the C	Complete rings in primary bronchi; plates, bars, and islands of cartilage with decreasing size	None
Clara cells	None	None	Increase in number with decreasing size of the branch

RESPIRATORY PORTION

Structure		Function	Location
Respiratory bronchiole			
Narrow, smallest of bronchioles, beginning of the respiratory portion		Air conduction, gas exchange	Distal-most branches of bronchioles
1. Ciliated simple cuboidal epithelium containing Clara cells: Cuboidal cells with apical dome-like projections		1. Condition inhaled air, capture particles and propel them upward, secrete surface-active agents and antimicrobial products	1. Luminal lining
2. Several alveoli: Directly arise from the bronchiole		2. Gas exchange	2. Scattered throughout the length of the bronchiole, increase in number distally
Alveolar ducts			
3. Extended air passageway from respiratory bronchiole		3. Conduct air from respiratory bronchiole to alveolar sacs	3. Distal to respiratory bronchioles
4. Series of alveoli open to a common channel		4. Gas exchange	4. Line the air channel

(continued)

RESPIRATORY PORTION (continued)

Structure		Function	Location
Alveolar ducts			
5. Knob-like structures cap the alveolar edge		5. Provide limited structural support, protection and contraction of alveolar ducts	5. Alveolar edges facing the duct
a. Cuboidal epithelium			a. In contact with air
b. Smooth muscle cells			b. Deep to epithelium
Alveolar sac			
6. Common space into which a cluster of alveoli open		6. Terminal air conduit to the terminal clusters of alveoli	6. Distal to alveolar ducts
Alveolus			
Spherical terminal air space composed of:			
7. Simple squamous epithelium		7. Gas exchange, lubrication of alveolar lining	7. Luminal lining
c. Type I alveolar cells (pneumocytes): Squamous cells		c. Gas exchange across the cell	c. 95% of the alveolar luminal lining
d. Type II alveolar cells (pneumocytes): Cuboidal cells		d. Surfactant production	d. Scattered throughout alveolar wall, often at septal junctions

Structure	Function	Location
Alveolus		
e. Macrophages: Irregular-shaped cells, often with carbon particles	e. Phagocytosis of dust, cell debris, pathogens	e. Scattered in alveolar septa, occasionally in alveolar space
8. Thin connective tissue layer carrying:	8. Structural and functional support	8. Under the epithelium
f. Continuous capillaries	f. Gas exchange across the cell	f. Share basement membrane with type I alveolar cells

Additional Concepts

- **Surfactant:** Reduces the surface tension in alveoli and prevents them from collapsing and closing the air space. Premature infants with insufficient surfactant production are at increased risk of respiratory distress syndrome due to the inability to expand the collapsed alveoli.
- **Alveolar septum (septal wall):** A wall formed by two or more alveoli abutting each other, sharing a common connective tissue and capillaries in the middle. Hence, the alveolar septum is composed of two alveolar epithelial linings and connective tissue in the middle (FIG. 10-1).
- **Alveolar pores:** The openings in alveolar septa through which air can pass between alveolar spaces, allowing aeration of alveoli distal to obstruction.
- **Blood-air barrier:** A set of structures the gas crosses between the air space and blood during the gas exchange process. The barrier is composed of the cytoplasm of the type I alveolar cell, the cytoplasm of the capillary endothelial cell, and the basement membrane shared between the two cells (FIG. 10-2).
- **Segmental branching of the bronchi:** Allows pathologic portions of the lungs to be removed without affecting other segments of the bronchial tree.

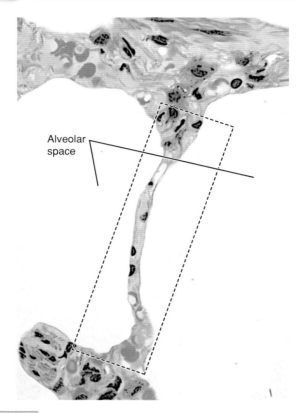

Alveolar
space

Figure 10-1. Interalveolar septum.

Clinical Significance

- **Anthracosis:** Accumulation of carbon dusts or particles in the lung tissues leading to varying degrees of blackened appearance of the lungs. Inhaled carbon dust particles (black) are engulfed by macrophages in the lungs. Some of these macrophages are removed, but some remain in the stroma of the lungs. Most urban dwellers exhibit some amount of anthracosis. Heavy smokers and coal miners exhibit more extensive anthracosis, and in severe

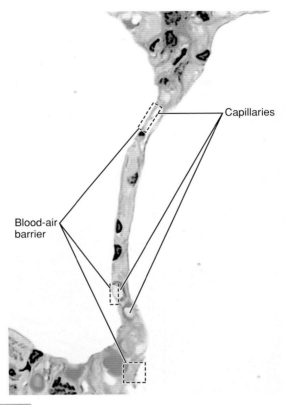

Figure 10-2. Blood-air barrier.

cases, it may progress to pneumoconiosis as the result of inflammation, fibrosis, and necrosis of the lung.

- **Emphysema:** Permanent enlargement of air space as the result of alveolar destruction and subsequent reduction of available surface area for gas exchange. Most common cause is prolonged exposure to noxious agents such as cigarette smoke.

Urinary System | 11

INTRODUCTION

Composed of two kidneys, two ureters, the urinary bladder, and the urethra, the urinary system plays a critical role in blood filtration, maintenance of fluid homeostasis, regulation of blood pressure, erythrocyte formation, and vitamin D conversion to an active form. Functionally, the urinary system is subdivided into the excretory portion (nephrons), responsible for blood filtration and production of urine, and the collecting portion (collecting ducts, calyces, ureter, bladder, and urethra), which receives, transports, and temporarily stores formed urine until excretion.

THE URINARY SYSTEM

KIDNEY		
Structure	Function	Location
Macroscopic features		
Bean-shaped, bilateral, red/ brown organs	Blood filtration, blood volume and pressure regulation, maintenance of body fluid homeostasis, production of erythropoietin, conversion of vitamin D to an active form	Retroperitoneal, vertebral level T12–L3 on either side of vertebral column (right kidney— slightly lower)
1. Capsule: Dense connective tissue	1. Protection	1. Outermost covering of the kidney

(continued)

KIDNEY (continued)

Structure		Function	Location
Macroscopic features			

2. Cortex: Red/brown outer layer

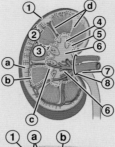

   a. Medullary rays: Linear striations extending from medulla

3. Medulla: Pink/lighter brown inner layer composed of:

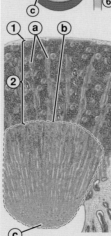

   b. Renal pyramids: Pyramidal pink/light brown lobes

   c. Renal papilla: Apex of the renal pyramid

   d. Renal columns: Extensions of cortical tissue in the medulla

4. Renal sinus: Space filled with calyces and adipose tissue

Function column:

2. Various stages of urine formation

   a. Collection, drainage, concentration of urine

3. Urine concentration

   b. Regulation and maintenance of hyperosmolality of the interstitium

   c. Drainage of formed urine into minor calyx

   d. Extension of the cortical tissue into the medulla

4. Contain, protect, and insulate calyces, blood vessels

Location column:

2. Deep to capsule

   a. Throughout cortex in radial arrangement

3. Deep to cortex

   b. Several throughout medulla

   c. Tip/apex of the renal pyramid: Extend out into renal sinus

   d. In the medulla, in between the renal pyramids

4. Center of the kidney

Structure	Function	Location
Macroscopic features		
5. Minor calyx: Short, small, cup-like structures each abutting renal papilla	5. Collect formed urine from collecting ducts	5. In renal sinus, at each renal papilla
6. Major calyx: Short, bigger tubular structure	6. Collect urine from minor calyces	6. In renal sinus, distal to minor calyces
7. Renal pelvis: Funnel-shaped drainage	7. Collect urine from major calyces and drain into ureter	7. Renal sinus, near hilum
8. Renal hilum: Indentation, depression	8. Ureter, vessels, and nerves enter and exit the kidney	8. Medial surface of the kidney
Microscopic features: Nephron		
1. Renal corpuscle: Spherical structures	1. Filtration of blood	1. Throughout renal cortex
a. Glomerulus: Loops of fenestrated capillaries	a. Flow of blood; initial passage of filtrate through fenestrae and endothelial cell	a. Inside the renal corpuscle
b. Visceral layer of Bowman capsule: Podocytes	b. Allow filtrate to pass between filtration slit to enter the urinary space	b. Coating outside of the glomerular capillary loops

(continued)

KIDNEY (continued)

Structure	Function	Location

Microscopic features: Nephron

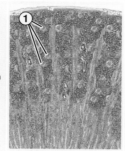

c. Parietal layer of Bowman capsule: Simple squamous epithelium

c. Containment of the filtrate

c. Outermost layer of the renal corpuscle

d. Urinary space

d. Reception, storage of filtrate

d. Between the visceral and parietal layers of Bowman capsule

e. Vascular pole

e. Entry and exit point for afferent and efferent arterioles

e. Opposite the urinary pole

f. Urinary pole

f. Filtrate in urinary space enter the PCT

f. Beginning of the PCT

2. Proximal convoluted tubule (PCT): Simple cuboidal epithelium with larger, eosinophilic cells and "fuzzy" luminal border (brush border)

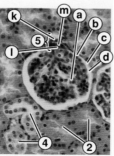

2. Majority of NaCl, fluid resorption; resorb amino acids, sugars, polypeptides; endocytose large peptides

2. Throughout renal cortex: More toward medulla

3. Loop of Henle

3. Concentration of urine

3. Begin and end in the renal cortex, but the loop extends into the medulla

Structure		Function	Location
Microscopic features: Nephron			
g. Thick descending limb: Simple cuboidal epithelium, permeable to water, impermeable to salt		g. Similar to PCT, but to a lesser extent	g. Cortex and medulla
h. Thin descending limb: Simple squamous epithelium		h. Resorb water, increase filtrate osmolality, impermeable to NaCl	h. Medulla
i. Thin ascending limb: Simple squamous epithelium		i. Resorb NaCl, impermeable to water, maintain the hyperosmotic interstitium	i. Medulla
j. Thick ascending limb: Simple cuboidal epithelium, permeable to NaCl, impermeable to water		j. Resorb NaCl, Ca^{2+}, Mg^{2+}	j. Medulla and cortex
4. Distal convoluted tubule (DCT): Simple cuboidal epithelium		4. Resorb Na^+, bicarbonate ions; secrete K^+, ammonium	4. Throughout renal cortex: More in the superficial potion

(continued)

KIDNEY (continued)		
Structure	**Function**	**Location**

Microscopic features: Nephron

5. Juxtaglomerular (JG) apparatus	5. Blood pressure regulation	5. Vascular pole of each renal corpuscle
k. Macula densa: Accumulation of thin, columnar cells within DCT	k. Monitor Na$^+$ concentration in the forming urine, regulate glomerular filtration rate (GFR) and release of renin from JG cells	k. Wall of the DCT in contact with lacis cells
l. JG cells: Smooth muscle cells of the afferent arteriole	l. Secrete renin in response to decreased blood volume/pressure	l. Wall of the afferent arteriole in contact with lacis cells
m. Lacis cells: Thin spindle cells	m. Structural support; phagocytose cellular debris, residues	m. Between macula densa and JG cells
6. Collecting tubules, ducts: Simple cuboidal to columnar epithelium	6. Urine concentration, acid-base balance regulation	6. Cortex and medulla

Additional Concepts

- **Excretory portion of the urinary system:** Composed of approximately 2 million nephrons in each kidney that actively filter blood and produce urine.

- **Collecting portion of the urinary system:** Composed of the collecting tubules, ducts, minor and major calyces, renal pelvis, ureters, urinary bladder, and urethra.
- **Nephron:** Structural and functional unit of the kidney composed of the following segments (FIG. 11-1):
  - **Renal corpuscle:** Spherical structure made of glomerulus surrounded by a double-layered Bowman capsule where initial blood filtration occurs.
  - **Proximal convoluted tubule:** Much of resorption and secretion occurs here.
  - **Loop of Henle:** Where concentration of urine takes place.
  - **Distal convoluted tubule:** Where resorption, acid-base balance occurs.
  - **Juxtaglomerular apparatus:** Composed of macula densa of the DCT, JG cells of the afferent arteriolar smooth muscle, and lacis

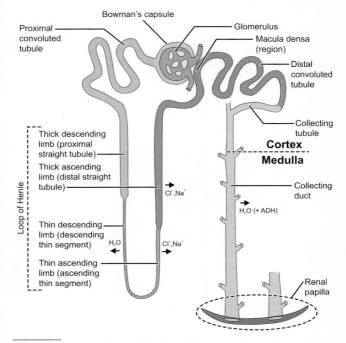

Figure 11-1. Nephron. (From Cui D. *Atlas of Histology.* Baltimore: Lippincott Williams & Wilkins, 2009:231.)

cells. Regulates blood volume and pressure via renin-angiotensin-aldosterone system.

- **Collecting tubules and ducts:** Though they belong to the collecting portion of the urinary system, urine concentration still takes place under the regulation of the posterior pituitary hormone, antidiuretic hormone (ADH)/vasopressin.
- **Glomerular filtration barrier:** Layers through which blood filtrate passes to enter the urinary space. Composed of glomerular endothelium, basement membrane, and podocyte filtration slits of the visceral layer of the Bowman capsule. The basement membrane in particular plays a critical role in restricting the movement of large proteins and charged molecules (FIG. 11-2).
- **Cortical nephrons:** Positioned closer to the capsule with the loop of Henle traveling only a short distance into the medulla. Hence, urine produced is not as heavily concentrated.
- **Juxtamedullary nephrons:** Positioned closer to the medulla with the loop of Henle traveling deep into the medulla. Hence, urine produced is more concentrated.
- **Renin-angiotensin-aldosterone system:** Regulates sodium homeostasis, glomerular filtration rate, and water resorption. In response to blood volume/pressure decrease and/or low sodium intake, juxtaglomerular cells of the juxtaglomerular apparatus secrete renin. Renin converts circulating angiotensinogen to angiotensin I, which is then converted to an active form, angiotensin II, in the lungs. Angiotensin II then stimulates aldosterone release from the adrenal zona glomerulosa. Aldosterone stimulates increased sodium and

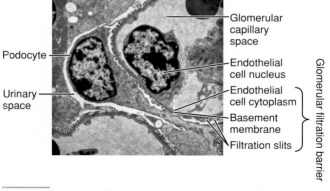

Figure 11-2. Glomerular filtration barrier. (From Eroschenko VP. *diFiore's Atlas of Histology with Functional Correlations*. 12th ed. Baltimore: Lippincott Williams & Wilkins, 2009:435.)

water resorption at the DCT and collecting ducts, thereby increasing blood volume and pressure.

- **Vasopressin (antidiuretic hormone):** A hormone released from the neurohypophysis (posterior pituitary) in response to reduced blood volume and increased plasma osmolality. ADH increases the water channel (aquaporin 2) assembly in the collecting tubules and ducts, allowing more water resorption and retention in the body. Pituitary tumors that cause reduced ADH production result in hypervolumic, hypo-osmotic urine formation and associated polyuria and polydipsia.

Clinical Significance

- **Urinalysis:** Performed to screen for the presence of microorganisms, crystals, blood cells (hematuria), protein (proteinuria), and other abnormal chemical composition and pH that may indicate renal disease.
- **Diabetic nephropathy:** Common complication in patients with diabetes mellitus. Characterized by compromised glomerular filtration with thickening of the glomerular basement membrane, atherosclerotic arterioles, and glomerular sclerosis, eventually resulting in renal insufficiency and/or failure.

BLOOD SUPPLY TO THE KIDNEY			
Structure		**Function**	**Location**
Blood supply			
1. Renal artery		1. Carry blood from the aorta to the kidney	1. Arises directly from either side of the abdominal aorta between vertebral levels L1–L2
2. Interlobar artery		2. Carry blood into each lobe of the kidney	2. Renal sinus and renal columns
3. Arcuate artery		3. Carry blood to the cortex–medulla boundary	3. Runs along the base of the renal pyramid

(continued)

BLOOD SUPPLY TO THE KIDNEY (continued)

Structure	Function	Location
Blood supply		
4. Interlobular artery	4. Carry blood to each lobule of the kidney	4. Runs perpendicular to arcuate artery toward the capsule
5. Afferent arteriole	5. Carry blood into the renal corpuscle	5. Vascular pole
6. Glomerulus	6. Take part in the initiation of blood filtration	6. Within the renal corpuscle
7. Efferent arteriole	7. Carry blood away from the renal corpuscle	7. Vascular pole
8. a. Peritubular capillaries	8. a. Pick up water and minerals resorbed from PCT, DCT, and collecting tubules and ducts	8. a. Cortex
b. Vasa recta	b. Pick up water and minerals resorbed from loop of Henle and collecting tubules and ducts	b. Renal pyramids of the medulla
9. Interlobular veins	9. Drain blood from peritubular capillaries	9. Run along the interlobular artery

Structure	Function	Location
Blood supply		
10. Arcuate veins	10. Drain blood from vasa recta and interlobular veins	10. Run along the base of the renal pyramid
11. Interlobar veins	11. Drain blood from arcuate veins	11. Renal sinus and renal columns
12. Renal veins	12. Drain blood from each lobe and carry it to inferior vena cava	12. Enter inferior vena cava at vertebral levels L1–L2

Clinical Significance

- **Lobar or lobular necrosis of the kidney:** Due to sharp, 90-degree angles of the arcuate and interlobular arteries, thrombi can easily lodge at the branching junctions. Because of the organization of the kidney blood supply (one interlobar artery supplying one lobe, one interlobular artery supplying one lobule), such blockage causes a sharply demarcated area of necrosis without disseminated impact on the rest of the kidney.

URETER		
Structure	Function	Location
Macroscopic features		
Long, pink, fleshy tube with a narrow lumen	Conduct urine from renal pelvis to the urinary bladder	Extends from renal pelvis to the urinary bladder; retroperitoneal

(continued)

URETER (continued)

Microscopic features

Composed of
three layers:

1. Mucosa

   a. Epithelium:
      Transitional
      epithelium

   b. Lamina pro-
      pria: Loose
      to dense
      connective
      tissue

2. Muscular
   layer: Smooth
   muscles

3. Serosa and
   adventitia:
   Loose con-
   nective
   tissue with
   and without
   mesothelium,
   respectively

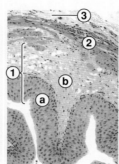

1. Line the
   lumen

   a. Line, pro-
      tect the
      mucosa,
      allow
      some dis-
      tension

   b. Protection
      and sup-
      port of
      epithe-
      lium

2. Peristalsis
   ensures
   directed flow
   of urine

3. Protection
   and adhe-
   sion of
   ureter to
   surrounding
   tissues

1. Innermost
   layer

   a. Directly
      in contact
      with the
      luminal
      content

   b. Deep to
      epithelium

2. Middle layer

3. Outermost
   layer

URINARY BLADDER

Structure		Function	Location
Macroscopic features			
Distensible organ; changes size and shape as it fills		Temporary urine storage, regulation of micturition	Pelvic cavity; posterior to pubic symphysis; anterior to rectum in males, uterus in females

Structure		Function	Location
Macroscopic features			
1. Two ureteric orifices		1. Urine entrance into the bladder. As bladder fills, openings are closed shut by bladder wall musculature.	1. Posterior wall of the bladder wall
2. Urethral orifice		2. Urine outlet	2. Inferior pole of the bladder
3. Trigone: Triangular region bounded by the three openings		3. Remain relatively unchanged during distension	3. Triangular region bounded by the three openings
Microscopic features			
Composed of three layers:			
4. Mucosa		4. Line the lumen	4. Innermost layer
a. Epithelium: Transitional epithelium		a. Line, protect, allow distension	a. In contact with the luminal content
b. Lamina propria: Loose to dense connective tissue		b. Protect and support epithelium	b. Deep to epithelium
5. Muscular layer: Smooth muscles		5. Peristalsis ensures directed flow of urine	5. Middle layer

	URINARY BLADDER (continued)		
Structure		**Function**	**Location**
6. Serosa and adventitia: Loose connective tissue with and without mesothelium, respectively		6. Protection and adhesion of ureter to surrounding tissues	6. Outermost layer

Additional Concepts

HISTOLOGIC LOOK-A-LIKES

	PCT	DCT	Collecting Tubules and Ducts
Tissue	Simple cuboidal epithelium	Simple cuboidal epithelium	Simple cuboidal to columnar epithelium
Lumen	Narrow; border is not clearly defined and "fuzzy"	Larger than PCT; border is more clearly defined than PCT	Same to larger than DCT; border is clearly defined
Cells	Large, eosinophilic cells with brush border; cell–cell borders are ill defined	Smaller than PCT cells; light pink–staining cytoplasm; ill-defined cell–cell border	Clear, pale-staining cuboidal to columnar cells; well-defined cell–cell borders

Clinical Significance

- **Autosomal dominant polycystic kidney disease:** Progressive formation and enlargement of cysts in the kidney and other organs that manifest clinical symptoms in the fourth decade of life. As the cysts overtake the kidney parenchyma, patients develop hypertension, renal insufficiency, and eventually renal failure.
- **Autosomal recessive (infantile/pediatric) polycystic kidney disease:** Formation of cysts in the collecting ducts and clinical presentation such as enlarged kidneys, abdominal mass, polyuria, and polydipsia in infancy and childhood.

Endocrine System | 12

INTRODUCTION

The endocrine system is composed of a number of organs, clusters of or individual cells that produce and secrete hormones into the bloodstream to signal distant target cells or organs. Most of the endocrine units derive from the lining epithelial invaginations that eventually lose their ducts and connections to the lining epithelium. Fenestrated capillaries are common stromal components that pick up, transport and deliver hormones.

THE ENDOCRINE SYSTEM

The pituitary is considered to be the master endocrine gland because its hormones have many target organs, including other endocrine organs.

PITUITARY GLAND/HYPOPHYSIS			
Structure		**Function**	**Location**
Macroscopic features			
Two distinct endocrine units:		Synthesis and release of nine hormones into bloodstream	Inferior to hypothalamus: In sella turcica of the sphenoid bone
1. Anterior pituitary (adenohypophysis/ anterior lobe): Pyramidal epithelioid cells arranged in ovoid clusters		1. Seven hormones: GH, prolactin, MSH, FSH, LH, ACTH, TSH	A fold of dura mater, diaphragma sellae, forms a roof over the pituitary gland

(continued)

PITUITARY GLAND/HYPOPHYSIS (continued)

Structure		Function	Location
Macroscopic features			
2. Posterior pituitary (neurohypophysis/ posterior lobe): Resembles neural tissue	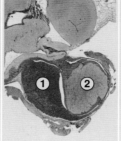	2. Two hormones: ADH (vasopressin), oxytocin	

Anterior pituitary/Adenohypophysis/Anterior lobe

Divided into three regions:	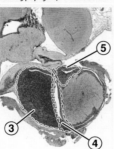	In response to hypothalamic hormones, synthesize and release appropriate hormones:	
3. Pars distalis: Consists of chromophobes and both chromophils		3. GH, prolactin, FSH, LH, ACTH, TSH	3. Majority of anterior pituitary
4. Pars intermedia: Consists of basophils and Rathke cysts	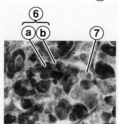	4. MSH	4. Small strip of glandular tissue between pars distalis and posterior pituitary
5. Pars tuberalis: Mostly basophils		5. FSH, LH	5. Extension of anterior pituitary surrounding infundibulum
Composed of three distinguishable endocrine cell types:			

Structure	Function	Location
Anterior pituitary/Adenohypophysis/Anterior lobe		
6. Chromophils	6.	6.
a. Acidophils: red to maroon staining cells	a. GH, prolactin	a. Pars distalis and pars tuberalis
b. Basophils: blue to purple staining cells	b. MSH, FSH, LH, ACTH, TSH	b. All three regions of anterior pituitary
7. Chromophobes: clear staining cells	7. Thought to be chromophils that have released all the secretory vesicles containing hormones	7. Pars distalis
Posterior pituitary/Neurohypophysis/Posterior lobe		
Divided into two regions	Hormones produced from supraoptic and paraventricular nuclei of hypothalamus are stored in axon terminals (Herring bodies) until appropriate stimuli triggers secretion	
8. Pars nervosa: Neural tissue: Neuropils, axon terminals, and pituicytes	8. Store and release ADH (vasopressin) and oxytocin	8. Majority of the posterior pituitary
9. Infundibulum: Composed of axons of the hypothalamic neurons	9. Connect pituitary to hypothalamus	9. Narrow stalk between hypothalamus and pituitary

(continued)

PITUITARY GLAND/HYPOPHYSIS (continued)

Structure	Function	Location
Posterior pituitary/Neurohypophysis/Posterior lobe		
Two distinguishable structures		
10. Herring bodies: Dilated axon terminals with neurosecretory vesicles	10. Store and release neurosecretory vesicles	10. Anucleate structures throughout pars nervosa
11. Pituicytes: Glial cells of the pituitary	11. Similar function as astrocytes: Structural and functional support to the neural components	11. Nucleated cells (oval) throughout pars nervosa

GH, growth hormone; MSH, melanocyte-stimulating hormone; FSH, follicle-stimulating hormone; LH, luteinizing hormone; ACTH, adrenocorticotropic hormone; TSH, thyroid-stimulating hormone; ADH, antidiuretic hormone.

Additional Concepts

- **Embryonic origin:** Adenohypophysis derives from the oral ectodermal invagination (Rathke pouch), whereas neurohypophysis derives from the diencephalon neural tissue down-growth, hence the histologic difference.
- **Hypothalamus:** Considered to be the master endocrine switch because it regulates the activity of the pituitary, the master endocrine gland
- **Blood supply:** Of functional significance, adenohypophysis does not have a direct blood supply; instead, it is supplied by the second capillary network of the hypophyseal portal system that first runs through the hypothalamic median eminence, carrying hypothalamic regulatory hormones to the adenohypophysis to influence its endocrine function (FIG. 12-1).

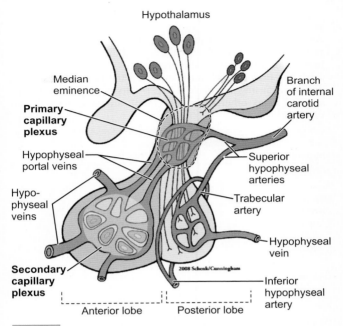

Figure 12-1. Blood supply to the pituitary gland.

MNEMONIC

GPA and My FLAT B

This phrase will help you remember the two types of chromophils of adenohypophysis and their hormone products:

Growth hormone and **P**rolactin from **A**cidophis.
MSH, **F**SH, **L**H, **A**CTH, and **T**SH from **B**asophi.

Clinical Significance

- **Pituitary adenomas:** Benign tumors of the anterior pituitary; may result in decreased or increased production of any of the pituitary hormones, causing wide variety and varying degrees of symptoms
- **Cushing disease:** Increased production of ACTH results in increased cortisol secretion by the adrenal glands, causing the characteristic pattern of weight gain in the trunk and face and other complex symptoms.

- **Gigantism:** Increased production of GH before the epiphyseal plates are calcified; results in above-average height.
- **Acromegaly:** Increased production of GH after the epiphyseal plates are calcified; results in enlarged and thickened facial bones, hands, and feet and visceral overgrowth.
- **Diabetes insipidus:** Tumors affecting the brain or neurohypophysis causing decreased ADH; results in polyuria, polydipsia, and many other signs and complications associated with dehydration.

ADRENAL GLAND		
Structure	**Function**	**Location**
Macroscopic features		
Paired, triangular glands covered with:		Positioned on top of each kidney
1. Capsule: Dense connective tissue	1. Coverage, protection, support	1. Superficial-most, protective layer
Organized into:	Synthesis and release of hormones into bloodstream	
2. Cortex: Slightly more cellular, outer layer	2. Steroid hormones: mineralocorticoids, glucocorticoids, gonadocorticoids	2. Deep to capsule
3. Medulla: Inner core containing loosely arranged chromaffin cells	3. Catecholamines	3. Core of the gland
Microscopic features		
Cortex is divided into three zones: Zona:	Synthesis and release of hormones:	

Structure	Function	Location
Microscopic features		
4. Glomerulosa: Small pyramidal cells in ovoid clusters	4. Mineralocorticoids: Primarily aldosterone: regulates Na^+, K^+, water balance in distal tubules of the nephron	4. Thin, superficial region of the cortex, immediately under the capsule
5. Fasciculata: Bigger, round cells with vacuolated cytoplasm arranged in long, straight cords	5. Glucocorticoids: Primarily cortisol; increases gluconeogenesis and glycogenesis	5. Thick middle region of the cortex
6. Reticularis: Smaller cells, in anastomosing cords	6. Gonadocorticoids: Primarily DHEA	6. Thin region in contact with medulla
Medulla:		
7. Chromaffin cells: Large, pale, modified postsynaptic neurons	7. Epinephrine, norepinephrine	7. Throughout medulla

Additional Concepts

Dual blood supply for the medulla:

- Arterial blood from medullary arterioles
- Venous blood from the cortex; allows cortical hormones to influence adrenal medullary structure and function

MNEMONIC

Get Facts Right: Men are Glued to Gonads

This phrase represents the adrenal cortical layers and corresponding hormone products:

Glomerulosa/**F**asciculata/**R**eticularis: **M**ineralocorticoids/**G**lucocorticoids/**Gonad**ocorticoids

Clinical Significance

- **Pheochromocytoma:** A tumor of chromaffin cells producing excess catecholamines, resulting in hypertension, anxiety, arrhythmias, digestive disfunction, etc.
- **Addison disease:** An adrenal insufficiency resulting from reduced production of steroid hormones from the adrenal cortex that causes symptoms such as hypotension, hyperpigmentation, fatigue, lightheadedness, weakness, and weight loss

THYROID GLAND		
Structure	**Function**	**Location**
Macroscopic features		
1. Right and left lobes connected by isthmus	1. Production, storage, and secretion of thyroid hormones T_3 and T_4 and secretion of calcitonin	1. Inferior to the thyroid cartilage, anterior to the trachea
2. Connective tissue capsule and septa	2. Surround the entire thyroid and separate parenchyma into lobules	2. Capsule surrounds the surface; septa irregularly extends into thyroid.
3. Spherical follicles of varying size filled with gelatinous colloid form the parenchyma	3. Storage of colloid, iodide; hormone production and secretion	3. Throughout thyroid parenchyma

Structure	Function	Location
Microscopic features		
4. Follicles composed of cuboidal to squamous follicular cells	4. Storage of colloid, iodide; production of hormones T_3, T_4; basal metabolism regulation	4. Lining of the follicles
5. Parafollicular cells (clear cells/C cells) in small groups or individual cells	5. Production of calcitonin; inhibit osteoclasts and decrease blood calcium level	5. Usually in between the follicles, sometimes in the follicular epithelium

Additional Concepts

HISTOLOGIC LOOK-A-LIKES

	Thyroid Gland	Active Mammary Gland
Parenchyma	Eosinophilic, colloid-filled follicles and no ducts	Vesicular appearance of lumen in dilated acini; areas of undilated acini and ducts are present
Stroma	Capsule on the surface; adipocytes and other connective tissue components are rare.	No capsule; adipocytes and other connective tissue components are present

Clinical Significance

- **Hyperthyroidism (toxic goiter/Graves disease):** Autoantibodies stimulate follicular cells to release excess amount of thyroid hormones resulting in thyroid hypertrophy (goiter), protrusion of the eyeballs, increased metabolism, weight loss, tachycardia, etc.
- **Hypothyroidism:** Reduced thyroid hormone production due to lack of iodine or autoantibodies that triggers apoptosis of follicular cells resulting in thyroid hypertrophy (goiter), weight gain, and mental and physical sluggishness.

PARATHYROID GLAND

Structure	Function	Location
Macroscopic features		
Four small glands composed of densely cellular parenchyma with connective tissue capsule and septa	Production and secretion of parathyroid hormone (PTH)	Posterior surface of the thyroid
Microscopic features		
1. Chief cells with clear cytoplasm and relatively large nuclei form the major component of the organ	1. Production and secretion of PTH; indirectly stimulate osteoclasts and increase blood calcium level	1. Throughout the organ in clusters or cords
2. Oxyphil cells: Larger, eosinophilic cytoplasm; small, dark nuclei	2. Unknown	2. Scattered throughout the organ in small groups or as individual cells
3. Adipocytes: Numbers increase with age	3. Fat storage	3. Scattered in small groups or as individual cells

Clinical Significance

- **Hypercalcemia:** Elevated blood calcium level commonly resulting from hyperparathyroidism. Complications include kidney stones, constipation, and osteitis fibrosa cystica.

PINEAL GLAND

Structure		Function	Location
Macroscopic features			
Small, fleshy ovoid neuroendocrine gland with occasionally visible macroscopic brain sands		Production and secretion of melatonin; regulate circadian rhythms	Posterior midline extension of the epithalamus
Microscopic features			
1. Pinealocytes: Modified neurons with ovoid nuclei and pale cytoplasm		1. Production and secretion of melatonin	1. Throughout the organ
2. Neuroglial cells (pineal astrocytes) resemble astrocytes		2. Support	2. Throughout the organ, more around capillaries
3. Brain sand (corpora arenacea): Dark, calcified bodies of varying size		3. Unknown	3. Randomly scattered

Additional Concepts

HISTOLOGIC LOOK-A-LIKES

	Parathyroid Gland	Pineal Gland	Prostate Gland
Parenchyma	Densely cellular organ, composed of chief cells and oxyphil cells, no calcified concretions	Resembles neural tissue with pinealocytes and glial cells; concretions (corpora arenacea) present	Exocrine glandular organization with ducts and distinct boundary between glands and stroma; concretions (corpora amylacea) present
Stroma	Scant stroma; adipocytes increase in number with age	Glial cells and neuropils	Mostly dense connective tissue

Clinical Significance

- **Medical imaging:** Pineal glands are easy to spot due to central location in the brain and radio-opaque calcifications on computed tomography and x-rays and serve as a useful landmark.

Male Reproductive System

13

INTRODUCTION

The male reproductive system consists of two testes, in which spermatozoa and male hormones are produced; a series of genital ducts that drain and deliver semen products to the urethra; accessory glands that secrete the majority of the fluid component of semen; and the penis, the copulatory organ. At puberty, an increase in sex hormones triggers the secondary male sex characteristics to develop and initiates sperm production in the testes. Sperm production is continuous and steady throughout the rest of adult males' lives.

THE MALE REPRODUCTIVE SYSTEM

TESTIS			
Structure		**Function**	**Location**
Macroscopic features			
Paired oval organ		Spermatozoa and male hormone production	Scrotal sac
1. Tunica vaginalis: Thin, delicate, double-layered serous membrane		1. Allowing movements of testis within scrotal sac and reducing friction	1. Anterolateral portion of each testis
2. Tunica albuginea: Dense connective tissue capsule		2. Surrounding and protecting the testes	2. Deep to tunica vaginalis

(continued)

TESTIS (continued)		
Structure	Function	Location

Macroscopic features

3. Septa: Extensions of the capsule into the parenchyma

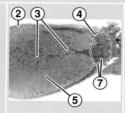

4. Mediastinum testis: Thickened dense connective tissue

3. Dividing testis parenchyma into lobules

4. Housing rete testis and forming a point of exit

3. Extend into the testis

4. Posterior thickening of the tunica albuginea

Microscopic features

5. Seminiferous tubules: Series of long, coiled tubules lined with germinal epithelium (resemble pseudostratified columnar epithelium)

   a. Sertoli cells: Tall, large, indistinct cell boundary; oval to triangular, euchromatic nuclei; distinct nucleoli

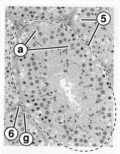

5. Production of germ cells, the spermatozoa

   a. Form tight junctions with each other, compartmentalize the tubule to basal and luminal sides, form testis-blood barrier, support spermatogenesis and spermiogenesis, remove debris

5. Within each lobule

   a. Throughout seminiferous tubules, extend the thickness of the tubule wall

Structure	Function	Location
Microscopic features		
b. Spermatogonia: Small, round cells, homogenous chromatin in the nuclei	b. Diploid stem cells that undergo mitosis, replenish stem cell population, and give rise to new spermatozoa	b. Basalmost portion of the seminiferous tubules below the Sertoli cell tight junctions
c. Primary spermatocytes: Larger cells with distinct thread-like chromosomes	c. Diploid cells undergoing meiosis I	c. Above the Sertoli cell tight junctions
d. Secondary spermatocytes: Smaller cells often in metaphase, difficult to identify due to short duration of meiosis II	d. Haploid products of meiosis I	d. Closer to the lumen
e. Spermatids: Varying morphology	e. Haploid products of meiosis II, undergoing spermiogenesis	e. Approach the lumen

(continued)

TESTIS (continued)		
Structure	**Function**	**Location**

Microscopic features

f. Sperma-tozoa: Elongated, condensed nuclei, fla-gella	f. Final product of sper-matogen-esis	f. Present in the lumen of semi-niferous tubules and in epididy-mis
6. Stroma: Connective tissue between seminiferous tubules	6. Support seminifer-ous tubules	6. In between seminifer-ous tubules
g. Leydig cells: Elongated, polyhedral cells; round, euchromatic nuclei; numerous vesicles	g. Produce and release testoster-one	g. Through-out stroma
7. Rete testis: Series of irreg-ular channels lined by simple cuboidal epi-thelium	7. Channel for conducting spermato-zoa from straight tubules to efferent ducts	7. Medias-tinum testis

Additional Concepts

- **Spermatogenesis:** Process of meiosis in which spermatogonium undergoes mitosis to give rise to the primary spermatocytes that undergo meiosis I, producing two haploid secondary spermatocytes. Secondary spermatocytes undergo meiosis II to produce four haploid spermatids. Spermatids undergo the process of morphologic trans-formation called spermiogenesis in which the nuclei are condensed,

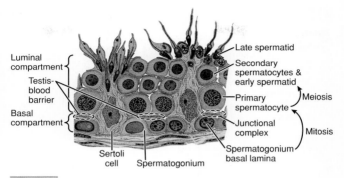

Figure 13-1. Seminiferous tubule: Spermatogenesis and testis-blood barrier. (From Ross MH, Pawlina W. *Histology: A Text and Atlas*. 6th ed. Baltimore: Lippincott Williams & Wilkins, 2009:791.)

the majority of the cytoplasm is shed, acrosome caps containing digestive enzymes form over the nuclei, and flagella are formed. Approximately 300 million sperm cells are produced daily (FIG. 13-1).

* **Testis-blood barrier:** Formed by tight junctions between Sertoli cells forming a physical boundary between the basal and luminal compartments of the seminiferous tubules. As spermatogenesis progresses, genetically different, haploid spermatocytes are moved into the luminal compartment of the seminiferous tubules and become isolated and protected from the immune system (see FIG. 13-1).

GENITAL DUCTS			
Structure		**Function**	**Location**
Epididymis			
1. Comma-shaped structure made of a long coiled tube		1. Storage, maturation, transport of spermatozoa	1. Posterior surface of the testis
a. Pseudostratified columnar epithelium		a. Absorption and secretion of fluid, phagocytosis of cell debris	a. Lines the lumen

(continued)

GENITAL DUCTS (continued)

Structure		Function	Location
b. Stereocilia: Long microvilli projecting into the lumen from the epithelial cells	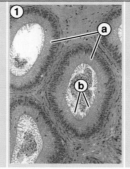	b. Increase surface area	b. Extend from the epithelial cell surface into the lumen

Vas (ductus) deferens

Structure		Function	Location
2. Paired, long, thick, muscular tube	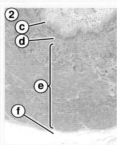	2. Conduct spermatozoa from epididymis to the ejaculatory ducts	2. Extend from the tail of epididymis to the prostate gland
c. Pseudostratified columnar epithelium with stereocilia		c. Limited absorption, secretion	c. Lines the lumen
d. Lamina propria: Connective tissue		d. Support the epithelium	d. Under the epithelium
e. Thick smooth muscle layers		e. Contract to propel spermatozoa	e. Middle layer
f. Adventitia: Loose connective tissue		f. Carry blood supply, adhere to surrounding structures	f. Outermost layer; blend in with surrounding connective tissues

Structure		Function	Location
Ejaculatory ducts			
3. Continuation of vas deferens within the prostate gland g. Pseudostratified columnar epithelium h. Connective tissue blends in with that of the prostate		3. Mix and transport spermatozoa and seminal vesicle secretions into the prostatic urethra	3. Obliquely traverse prostate from superior-posterior entrance of the vas deferens to central mid-point of the prostatic urethra

Additional Concepts

- **Ideal temperature for spermatogenesis:** 2°C to 3°C below body temperature. Elevated testicular temperature may cause infertility. Cooler temperature is maintained by the pampiniform venous plexus of the scrotum and spermatic cord that cool the arterial blood as it travels toward the testis. Cremaster muscles in the spermatic cord contract and relax to pull the testes closer or away from the body to maintain the steady temperature. Dartos muscles of the scrotum also contract in cold temperature to reduce heat loss.
- **Path of spermatozoa:** Seminiferous tubules → straight tubules (tubuli recti) → rete testis → efferent tubules → epididymis → vas deferens → ejaculatory ducts → prostatic urethra → membranous urethra → penile urethra
- **Vasectomy:** A relatively simple outpatient surgical procedure for male sterilization that involves cutting into the scrotum to isolate vasa deferentia and cutting them to ensure no spermatozoa can reach the distal ducts. The volume of semen is usually unaffected by the procedure, but no sperm cells are present in the ejaculate.

ACCESSORY GLANDS

Structure		Function	Location

Seminal vesicles

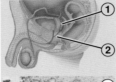

1. Paired glands composed of coiled secretory tubules

   a. Mucosal lining varies from simple to pseudostratified columnar epithelium

   b. Lamina propria: Thin, loose connective tissue

   c. Muscularis layer: Smooth muscles

1. Production of milky seminal fluid contributing 70% of the volume of semen

   a. Production of fructose-rich secretion

   b. Support the epithelium

   c. Contract to expel secretions into the ejaculatory ducts

1. Posterior wall of the bladder

   a. Lumen

   b. Under the epithelium

   c. Outside of the lamina propria

Prostate gland

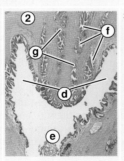

2. Oval to pyramidal organ

   d. Ejaculatory ducts: Continuation of vas deferens within the prostate

2. Contribute 25% to 30% of the volume of semen

   d. Deliver spermatozoa and seminal vesicle secretions to prostatic urethra

2. Inferior to urinary bladder

   d. Traverse prostate obliquely from superior-lateral to midportion of the prostatic urethra

Structure		Function	Location
Prostate gland			
e. Prostatic urethra: Portion of the urethra traversing the prostate		e. Conduct urine during micturition and semen during ejaculation	e. Midline of prostate from urinary bladder to membranous urethra
f. Prostatic glands: Compound tubuloacinar glands, simple to pseudostratified columnar epithelium		f. Secrete clear, slightly alkaline fluid	f. Throughout prostate
g. Prostatic concretions (corpora amylacea): Round, calcified acellular structures		g. No known function, increase in number with age	g. Throughout the lumen of the prostate glands

Additional Concepts

Prostatic zones:

- **Central zone:** Areas of the prostate immediately surrounding ejaculatory ducts containing some prostate glands. Rarely affected by inflammation or carcinomas
- **Peripheral zone:** Areas surrounding the central zone and posterolateral portions of the prostate containing most of the prostate glands. Most affected by prostatic carcinomas and inflammation
- **Transitional zone:** Small areas surrounding the prostatic urethra containing small amounts of prostate glands and some mucous glands. Site of prostate gland hyperplasia that causes benign prostatic hyperplasia (BPH)
- **Periurethral zone:** Areas anterolateral to the prostatic urethra that may be affected in later stage of BPH, further compressing the urethra and restricting urine flow

- **Fibromuscular zone:** Superior anterior strip-like region composed of dense irregular connective tissue, intermixed smooth muscle fibers, and little to no prostatic glands

Clinical Significance

- **BPH:** Almost always occurs in the transitional zone. Due to its proximity to the prostatic urethra, hyperplasia in this zone constricts the urethra, resulting in difficulty associated with urination. BPH occurs in a large percentage of the aging male population. Treatments vary from noninvasive medications that relax smooth muscles of the prostate to various surgical options to obliterate or remove the hypertrophic areas of prostate.
- **Prostatic carcinoma:** Almost always arises from the peripheral zone and is one of the most common cancers in the male. Due to the distance of the peripheral zone from the prostatic urethra, prostatic carcinoma does not affect urination until in the later stage after the tumor has reached a large size. Prostate-specific antigen (PSA) testing increases the early detection of prostatic carcinoma.

PENIS			
Structure		**Function**	**Location**
Macroscopic features			
Composed of three cylindrical erectile tissues		Urination and copulation	External genitalia
1. Tunica albuginea: Dense connective tissue capsule		1. Surround each erectile cylinder, form a capsule	1. Outside of each erectile cylinder
2. Corpora cavernosa: Paired erectile cylinders		2. Fill with blood to achieve erection	2. Dorsum of the penis
3. Corpus spongiosum: Single erectile cylinder		3. Fill with blood to achieve erection	3. Ventral midline of the penis
a. Glans penis: Terminal dilatation of corpus spongiosum		a. Form the dilated tip of the penis	a. Tip of the penis

Structure	Function	Location
Microscopic features		
4. Erectile tissues: Irregular, cavernous spaces lined with endothelium	4. Fill with blood to achieve erection	4. Throughout corpora cavernosa and corpus spongiosum
5. Penile urethra: Lined with pseudostratified columnar epithelium	5. Conduct urine and semen	5. In the middle and through the length of corpus spongiosum
6. Glands of Littre: Series of small, mucous-secreting glands	6. Secrete mucus into the penile urethra	6. Scattered throughout corpus spongiosum and open into penile urethra

Additional Concepts

- **Penile erection:** Occurs through parasympathetic stimulation that relaxes smooth muscles of the erectile tissues and dilation of arteries that deliver blood into the erectile bodies. As the cavernous spaces within the corpora cavernosa and corpus spongiosum fill with blood, the tissues compress the venous vessels against the tunica albuginea, therefore preventing blood drainage and achieving erection.
- **Termination of erection:** Sympathetic stimulation initiates contraction of smooth muscles of the erectile tissues and arteries, decreasing blood flow into the erectile tissues. Reduced pressure releases compression on the veins, allowing drainage of excess blood.

Clinical Significance

- **Erectile dysfunction:** An inability to achieve and/or maintain penile erection that may result from a multitude of causes ranging from psychological issues and blood pressure–related conditions to parasympathetic nerve damage. The active ingredient of Viagra enhances the smooth muscle relaxation within erectile tissues by increasing the effect of nitrogen oxide. In case of nerve damage, Viagra has no curative effect on achieving erection.

HISTOLOGIC LOOK-A-LIKES

	Rete Testis	Epididymis	Seminal Vesicles
Epithelia	Simple cuboidal epithelium, may resemble pseudostratified columnar epithelium in crowded areas, no stereocilia	Pseudostratified columnar epithelium with stereocilia	Varies from simple to pseudostratified columnar epithelium, no stereocilia
Mucosal folds	Moderate	Little to none	Extensive
Surrounding structures	Dense irregular connective tissue of the mediastinum testis, separating rete testes from each other. Nearby seminiferous tubules may be visible	Epididymis loops in various planes of section are present in close proximity. Small amount of connective tissue is present in between	One or more groups of highly folded mucosa are found surrounded and separated by a moderate amount of connective tissue

Female Reproductive System

14

INTRODUCTION

The female reproductive system consists of two ovaries, two uterine tubes, the uterus, the vagina, external genitalia, and mammary glands of the breasts. At puberty, increased female sex hormones induce the development of secondary sexual characteristics such as hyperplasia of the mammary glands and initiate regular ovarian and menstrual cycles. Under the influence of pituitary hormones, ovaries ovulate one oocyte per cycle and produce hormones that regulate the uterine lining to prepare for implantation in case of successful fertilization. In the absence of fertilization, the ovarian hormones decline and induce shedding of the uterine lining, which results in menstruation. Near the fifth decade of life, the ovarian and menstrual cycles end at menopause.

THE FEMALE REPRODUCTIVE SYSTEM

OVARIES		
Structure	**Function**	**Location**
Layers		
Paired oval to almond-shaped, gray to pink organs	Gametogenesis and hormone production	Retroperitoneal in pelvic cavity on either side of the uterus
1. Cortex: More cellular, pink to gray layer containing follicles of varying size	1. Site of oogenesis and ovulation, hormone production	1. Outer layer of the ovary

(continued)

OVARIES (continued)		
Structure	Function	Location

Layers

a. Germinal epithelium: Simple cuboidal to squamous mesothelium	a. Cover the outside of the ovary	a. Outermost layer
b. Tunica albuginea: Layer of dense irregular connective tissue	b. Form a protective capsule	b. Deep to germinal epithelium
c. Stroma: Cell-dense connective tissue	c. Provide supportive role for growing follicles; some differentiate into theca interna and externa cells	c. Throughout cortex
d. Follicles: Spherical structures of varying size	d. Support growth of oocyte and prepare for ovulation	d. Throughout cortex
2. Medulla: Vascular, inner layer	2. Delivery of vascular and neural supplies	2. Inner, central portion of the ovary

General features of the follicles

e. Oocytes: Large, pale-staining cells with large nuclei	e. Complete meiosis with follicular growth	e. Within the follicle, usually in the center

Structure		Function	Location
General features of the follicles			
f. Zona pellucida: Thick acellular layer surrounding oocyte		f. Form a protective shell around the oocyte	f. Immediately outside of the oocyte
g. Flat follicular cells or cuboidal granulosa cells		g. Protect and support the growing oocyte	g. Outside of the zona pellucida
h. Theca interna: Rounded stromal-driven cell layer		h. Secrete estrogen precursors	h. Outside of the granulosa cell layer, separated by a thin basement membrane
i. Theca externa: Spindle-shaped stromal cells and smooth muscle cells forming a capsule-like layer		i. Form a capsule-like structure, contract during ovulation	i. Outside of the theca interna; boundary is indistinct
j. Antrum: Fluid-filled space within granulosa cell layer		j. Fill with fluid, liquor folliculi, build pressure within the follicle, deliver nutrients	j. Within secondary follicles and Graafian follicles

(continued)

OVARIES (continued)

Structure		Function	Location

General features of the follicles

k. Corona radiata: Collection of granulosa cells that surround oocytes in Graafian follicles		k. Surround the oocyte	k. Outside of zona pellucida in Graafian follicles
l. Cumulus oophorus: Collection of granulosa cells		l. Connect the oocyte and corona radiata to the rest of the granulosa cells	l. Between the corona radiata and the rest of the granulosa cells

Types of follicles

3. Primordial follicle: Smallest, single layer of follicular cells surrounding a small oocyte without zona pellucida		3. Contain oocytes arrested in meiosis I	3. Cortical stroma near the tunica albuginea
4. Unilaminar primary follicles: Slightly bigger oocyte with zona pellucida surrounded by a single layer of cuboidal follicular (granulosa) cells		4. Contain and support growing oocytes	4–6. Follicles move deeper within the cortex as they grow in size to get closer to the blood supply in the medulla

Structure	Function	Location

General features of the follicles

5. Multilaminar primary follicles: Growing oocyte, surrounded by more than one layer of cuboidal granulosa cells; theca interna forms

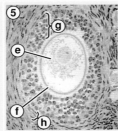

5. Contain and support growing oocytes; granulosa cells undergo mitosis, contributing to growing size of the follicle

6. Secondary (antral) follicles: Contain atria, fluid-filled spaces; theca interna and externa are seen

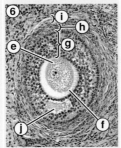

6. Contain and support growing oocytes, start to accumulate fluid to deliver nutrients to all cells within the enlarging follicle, produce estrogen

7. Graafian follicles: Large, single antrum, corona radiata, cumulus oophorus, distinct theca interna and externa

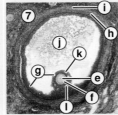

7. Contain and support oocytes that completed meiosis I and were arrested in metaphase II, build pressure within the follicle, increase production of estrogen, prepare for ovulation

7. Move closer to the tunica albuginea with increasing size and protrude out into the peritoneal cavity immediately before ovulation

(continued)

OVARIES (continued)

Structure		Function	Location
Corpus luteum			
Yellow, relatively large and convoluted structure that forms after ovulation by the remaining cells of the follicle		Production and secretion of estrogen and progesterone	At the site of ovulation
1. Granulosa lutein cells: Form the bulk of the corpus luteum; derived from the granulosa cells of the follicle; enlarged, polygonal cells with abundant cytoplasm and large, euchromatic nuclei		1. Production and secretion of estrogen and progesterone, conversion of sex hormone precursors	1. Throughout corpus luteum
2. Theca lutein cells: Derived from theca interna, much smaller, oval to spindle-shaped cells		2. Production of progesterone and androgens	2. Periphery and in between the folds of granulosa lutein cells of the corpus luteum
Corpus albicans			
Small, white, firm structure; resembles dense irregular connective tissue	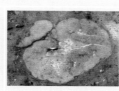	Remnant of corpus luteum degradation	Throughout ovarian cortex; numbers increase with age

Additional Concepts

- **Oogenesis:** Occurs during early fetal development. At birth, approximately 600,000 to 800,000 oocytes are present in primordial follicles. No additional oogenesis occurs. All oocytes remain arrested in the early stage of meiosis I until puberty. The majority of the primordial follicles are lost through atresia, a process of degradation and resorption, and only about 400 ova are ovulated in a lifetime.

- **Meiosis:** A long process in oocytes. As the follicles start to grow at puberty, oocytes complete meiosis I immediately before ovulation, resulting in one much bigger haploid oocyte and a much smaller polar body, which often degrades. The oocyte immediately enters meiosis II but is arrested at metaphase II. Unless fertilization occurs by a sperm cell, meiosis II will not complete and the oocyte undergoes degradation within 24 hours of ovulation.

- **Fertilization:** Occurs when a sperm successfully penetrates through the corona radiata and zona pellucida, injecting its haploid nuclear content into the oocyte. At this time, the oocyte completes meiosis II, again resulting in one big daughter cell and a much smaller polar body. The nuclear content of the ovum and the sperm fuse to form a genetically unique zygote, complete with 46 chromosomes, half from the ovum and the other half from the sperm.

- **Germinal epithelium** in the ovaries is a misnomer. The mesothelial lining of the ovarian surface was initially thought to be the site of oogenesis; hence, it was named germinal epithelium. Later, the true origin of the oocytes was identified to be within the ovarian cortex; however, the surface lining epithelium continues to be designated as germinal epithelium. The germinal epithelium of testes refers to the wall of the seminiferous tubules; thus, it is not a misnomer in the male.

- **Ovarian cycle:** Begins with follicle-stimulating hormone (FSH) from the pituitary that induces follicular growth. As the follicles grow, they secrete an increasing amount of estrogen, which stimulates uterine endometrial glandular proliferation and thickening. Once the circulating estrogen reaches a threshold, it triggers leuteinizing hormone (LH) release from the pituitary. LH triggers ovulation to take place, after which the remnant of the Graafian follicle involutes and forms a corpus luteum. The corpus luteum secretes progesterone in addition to estrogen. Progesterone induces the uterine endometrial glands to secrete nutrient-rich products in preparation for possible arrival and implantation of the fertilized conceptus. In the absence of pregnancy, the corpus luteum undergoes involution 10 to 12 days after ovulation and causes a decline in circulating estrogen and progesterone levels. In response, the endometrial lining is shed and the menstrual phase ensues. If a conceptus successfully implants in the endometrial lining, it starts to secrete human chorionic gonadotrophin (hCG), which stimulates the corpus luteum to hypertrophy and continue to secrete its hormones, preventing the shedding of the endometrial lining along with the conceptus. The corpus luteum continues to function for up to 8 weeks into pregnancy until the placenta produces enough estrogen and progesterone on its own; at this point, the corpus luteum starts to degrade, but it may persist throughout the duration of pregnancy.

UTERUS

Structure		Function	Location
Macroscopic features			
Pear-shaped pelvic organ		Support the implantation and development of the conceptus	Retroperitoneal pelvic cavity, between urinary bladder and rectum
1. Fundus: Dome-shaped anterior-superior portion		1. Expand to allow fetal growth	1. Anterior, superior portion of the uterus
2. Body: Triangular main portion		2. Most common site for implantation	2. Inferior to the fundus and the uterine tube openings
3. Cervix: Tapered, narrow inferior portion		3. Regulate passage of materials between the uterine space and the vagina	3. Inferior to the body
a. Cervical canal: Narrow opening through the cervix		a. Passage of menstrual products, conceptus, semen	a. Run vertically in the center of the cervix

Structure		Function	Location
Macroscopic features			
b. Internal os: Opening between uterine cavity and cervical canal		b. Regulate passage between uterine cavity and cervical canal	b. Opening into the uterine cavity
c. External os: Opening between cervical canal and vagina		c. Regulate passage between cervical canal and vagina	c. Opening into the vagina
d. Ectocervix: Cervical protrusion into vagina		d. Protect the inferior portion of the uterus	d. Inferior-most portion that evaginates into the vagina
e. Fornix: Recess around the ectocervix		e. Temporary storage of deposited semen	e. Recess around the ectocervix
Layers			
1. Endometrium: Mucosal layer with glands of varying morphology		1. Undergo cyclic changes in response to estrogen and progesterone	1. Inner layer of the uterus, in contact with uterine cavity
a. Stratum basale: Basal portion of endometrial glands; stromal cells are present		a. Source for regenerating and thickening stratum functionale	a. Deep layer, in contact with myometrium

(continued)

UTERUS (continued)

Structure		Function	Location
Layers			
b. **Stratum functionale:** Contain endometrial glands of varying morphology depending on hormones and stromal cells	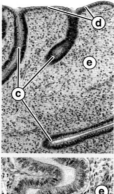	b. Proliferate and shed in response to hormones	b. Layer closer to the uterine cavity
c. **Endometrial glands:** Simple branched glands lined by simple columnar epithelium	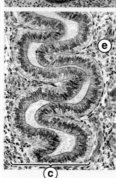	c. Lengthen and coil with growing endometrium, secrete nutrient-rich mucoid fluid	c. Throughout endometrium
d. **Endometrial lining epithelium:** Simple columnar epithelium		d. Line the uterine cavity	d. Surface layer in contact with uterine cavity
e. **Stroma:** Fairly cellular connective tissue containing small, uniform stromal cells		e. Support endometrial glands, transform into decidual cells in response to implantation	e. Throughout endometrium

Structure	Function	Location
Layers		
2. Myometrium: Thick layer of smooth muscles	2. Undergo hypertrophy and hyperplasia during pregnancy to accommodate growing fetus, undergo strong contractions during parturition	2. Middle layer of the uterus
3. Perimetrium: Mesothelial lining	3. Cover, cushion the uterus; reduce friction in movements against other organs	3. Posterior, superior, and small anterior portions of the uterus
Endometrium during menstrual cycle		
1. Proliferative phase: Thin endometrium gradually thickens with lengthening of straight, narrow, uniform glands in stratum functionale	1. At the end of menstrual phase, gradually thickens the endometrium under the influence estrogen	1. Days 5 to 14 in menstrual cycle which starts at the end of menstruation

(continued)

UTERUS (continued)

Structure	Function	Location

Endometrium during menstrual cycle

Structure	Function	Location
2. Early secretory phase: Endometrium thickens further; glands start to appear coiled, but have a smooth luminal outline; subnuclear vacuolation may be observed in glandular epithelium 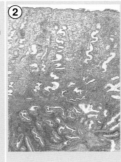	2. Under the influence of progesterone, glands start to secrete nutrient-rich mucoid fluid into the lumen and uterine cavity	2. Days 14 to 21 in menstrual cycle, immediately after ovulation
3. Late secretory phase: Thickest; glands are supercoiled; luminal outline is sessile and dilated; stromal edema is observed 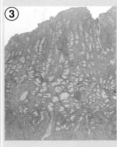	3. Under the influence of progesterone, secrete large amount of nutrient-rich fluid, prepare endometrium for possible implantation	3. Days 21 to 28 in menstrual cycle. Fertilized conceptus arrives in uterine cavity at approximately day 21 in menstrual cycle
4. Menstrual phase: Indistinct endometrial lining epithelium; stratum functionale loses structural integrity; erythrocytes are observed in the stroma and lumen	4. In the absence of estrogen and progesterone, stratum functionale is shed to prepare the endometrium for the next menstrual cycle	4. Days 0 to 5 in menstrual cycle

Structure		Function	Location
Cervix			
1. Mucosa: Thin; does not contain stratum functionale; does not shed at menstrual phase		1. Line the cervical canal, internal and external os	1. Innermost layer of the cervix
a. Cervical glands: Large, branched mostly mucous-secreting glands		a. Produce mucus of varying viscosity; increased production of more watery mucus near the ovulation aids in sperm migration into the uterine cavity	a. Throughout cervical mucosa
2. Muscularis: Smooth muscles are interspersed with large amount of collagen fibers. Elastic fibers increase near parturition		2. Continuous with myometrium, restrict expansion of the inferior uterus during pregnancy, allow fetal passage during parturition	2. Middle layer: Continuous with myometrium
3. Adventitia: Dense connective tissue		3. Secure and anchor the inferior portion of the uterus to the pelvic floor	3. Outermost layer of the cervix

(continued)

UTERUS (continued)

Structure	Function	Location

Cervix

4. Ectocervix: Lined with nonkeratinized stratified squamous epithelium

4. Cervical projection into the vagina

4. Bulges out into vaginal canal

b. Transformation zone: Site of abrupt epithelial transition from simple columnar epithelium of the cervical canal to the nonkeratinized stratified squamous epithelium of the ectocervix

b. Mark the epithelial transition and frequent site of metaplastic changes, hence monitored routinely during Pap smear procedures

b. In reproductively inactive women: Within cervical canal. In reproductively active women: Outside of external os

FALLOPIAN (UTERINE) TUBE

Structure	Function	Location

Macroscopic features

1. Infundibulum: Funnel-shaped distal expansion containing fimbriae

1. Drape over the ovaries to draw in the ovulated ovum

1. Distal-most portion of the fallopian tube, close proximity to the ovaries

2. Ampulla: Long, gradually narrowing tubular segment

2. Site of fertilization

2. Between the infundibulum and the isthmus

Structure		Function	Location
Macroscopic features			
3. Isthmus: Narrow, more muscular portion		3. Propel the ovum toward the uterus	3. Adjacent to the uterus
4. Uterine (intramural): Segment of the tubule traversing the uterine wall		4. Propel the ovum into the uterine cavity	4. Within the uterine wall
Histologic features			
1. Mucosa: Contains numerous longitudinal folds, greatest in infundibulum and decreases closer to the uterus		1. Folds increase surface area for contact with ovum	1. Lining of the fallopian tube
a. Lining: Ciliated simple columnar epithelium		a. Cilia create a current to conduct ovum toward the uterus	a. In contact with the lumen
b. Lamina propria: Loose connective tissue		b. Support lining epithelium	b. Deep to epithelium, core of the mucosal folds
2. Muscularis: Layer of smooth muscle cells, gets progressively thicker closer to uterus		2. Structural support and weak contraction to propel ovum toward the uterus	2. Middle layer: Continuous with the myometrium of uterus

FALLOPIAN (UTERINE) TUBE (continued)		
Structure	**Function**	**Location**
Histologic features		
3. Serosa: Mesothelial lining	3. Cover the surface of fallopian tubes	3. Outermost layer of fallopian tube, continuous with perimetrium

VAGINA		
Structure	**Function**	**Location**
Layers		
1. Mucosa: Contain numerous transverse folds	1. Receive penis during copulation, temporarily store semen, serve as a part of the birth canal during parturition	1. Innermost layer
a. Lining epithelium: Nonkeratinized stratified squamous epithelium	a. Form a protective lining	a. In contact with vaginal space
b. Lamina propria: Loose connective tissue, no glands	b. Support the epithelium	b. Deep to epithelium
2. Muscularis: Smooth muscles	2. Contract during copulation	2. Middle layer
3. Adventitia: Dense irregular connective tissue	3. Deliver vascular supply	3. Outermost layer, blends in with the surrounding connective tissue of the perineum

Clinical Significance

- **Pregnancy test:** Detects presence of hCG in the urine as early as 10 days of pregnancy.
- **Birth control:** A variety of hormone mimetics or antagonists are used to prevent pregnancy, many targeting the response of the endometrium to estrogen and progesterone to ensure the endometrium is not receptive to the conceptus.
- **Tubal ectopic pregnancy:** Results when the conceptus fails to enter the uterine cavity and instead implants in the fallopian tube. Due to thin mucosal lining, the placenta quickly invades into the thin muscularis layer as the conceptus grows. The muscular layer of the fallopian tube fails to accommodate the growing conceptus and eventually ruptures, causing massive bleeding from the compromised placental tissue. Such an event is an emergency that requires urgent surgery to remove the source of massive bleeding, the product of conception, and the fallopian tube.
- **Placenta accreta:** Occurs when growing fetal placenta invades the myometrial layer of the uterus, in which case removal of the placental tissue after birth is difficult, frequently resulting in a ruptured placenta that causes massive bleeding. Placenta accreta is associated with implantation of the conceptus near the cervix where the endometrium is thin and the stratum functionale is minimal to nonexistent.

MAMMARY GLANDS		
Structure	**Function**	**Location**
Macroscopic features		
1. Multiple lobes of exocrine glandular tissues	1. Produce and secrete milk	1. Throughout breast tissue
a. Compound tubuloacinar glands	a. Respond to estrogen, progesterone, and oxytocin	a. Surrounded by the dense connective and adipose connective tissue
b. Secretory alveoli: Simple cuboidal epithelium	b. Produce milk	b. Ends of the intralobular ducts

(continued)

MAMMARY GLANDS (continued)		
Structure	**Function**	**Location**

Macroscopic features

c. Intralobular ducts: Simple to stratified cuboidal epithelium		c. Drain alveoli	c. Throughout the lobules
d. Interlobular ducts: Simple to stratified cuboidal epithelium		d. Drain intralobular ducts	d. Within the septa
e. Lactiferous ducts: Stratified cuboidal to columnar epithelium		e. Drain interlobular ducts and open onto the nipple	e. Near the nipple
2. Dense irregular connective tissue: Form septa between lobes		2. Separate mammary gland lobes and lobules, anchor the breast tissue to the underlying muscle tissues	2. Throughout breast tissue
3. Adipose connective tissue		3. Store lipids, insulate and protect mammary glands	3. Throughout breast tissue

Inactive mammary glands

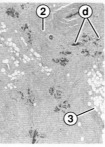

Small under-developed glands a. Small amount of inactive alveoli d. Interlobular ducts with narrow lumen 2. Abundant dense irregular connective tissue	Maintain potential to produce milk	Throughout breasts of adolescent and adult females who are not pregnant

Structure		Function	Location
Inactive mammary glands			
3. Abundant adipose connective tissue			
Active mammary gland			
Larger, dense and uniform glands		Glandular epithelium proliferates to produce more secretory alveoli and ductal systems	Pregnant female breasts
a. Abundant alveoli with dilated lumen			
b. Abundant intralobular ducts			
c. Distinct interlobular ducts			
2. Reduced dense connective tissue			
3. Reduced adipose connective tissue			
Lactating mammary gland			
Well developed, actively secreting glands		Actively secrete and transport milk to the nipple	Females after parturition
a. Abundant alveoli with dilated lumen are pushed up against each other			
2. Much reduced dense connective tissue			
3. Much reduced adipose connective tissue			

Clinical Significance

- **Breast cancer:** A variety of different types of cancer that arise from the mammary glands. Depending on which segment (duct or alveoli) and which type of cell the tumor originated from, the molecular profile and behavior of the tumor maybe distinct, hence requiring accurate diagnosis and specific treatment.
  - **DCIS (ductal carcinoma in situ):** Tumor that arises from the ductal components of the mammary glands; contained within the duct and has not broken through the basement membrane of the duct.
  - **LCIS (lobular carcinoma in situ):** Tumor that arises from the lobular (secretory) component of the mammary glands; contained within the alveolus and has not broken through the basement membrane.

HISTOLOGIC LOOK-A-LIKES

	Active Mammary Glands	Parotid Salivary Glands	Pancreas
Secretory units	Uniform size and shape of acinar (alveolar) secretory units lined with simple cuboidal epithelium, containing fairly good-sized lumen	Uniform size and shape of serous acinar (alveolar) secretory units lined with simple cuboidal epithelium, but lumens are small and indistinct	Uniform size and shape of serous acinar (alveolar) secretory units lined with simple cuboidal epithelium. Lumens are small and indistinct. Pale-staining islets of Langerhans are unique to pancreas
Ducts	Intra- and inter-lobular ducts are stratified cuboidal epithelium	Intercalated ducts are simple cuboidal epithelium. Presence of striated ducts is unique to salivary glands	Most ducts are simple cuboidal epithelium. No striated ducts
Surrounding structures	Dense irregular connective tissue surrounds each lobule; intermixed adipose connective tissues are observed	Thin connective tissue septa separate lobules; adipose connective tissue is uncommon	Thin connective tissue septa separate lobules; adipose connective tissue within the gland is uncommon

	Lactating Mammary Glands	Thyroid	Lungs
Secretory units	Areas of simple cuboidal epithelium–lined alveoli with large lumens with milk that appears dusty intermixed with areas that resemble active mammary glands are seen	Spherical follicles lined with simple cuboidal to simple squamous epithelia contain homogenous, eosinophilic colloids in the lumen. Pale-staining parafollicular cells are observed	Spherical alveoli lined with simple squamous epithelium are observed without any staining in the air space
Ducts	Much more dilated and elaborate ducts are lined by stratified cuboidal epithelium	No ducts are present	Respiratory, terminal bronchioles with simple cuboidal epithelia and bronchi with cartilage may be observed
Stroma	Thin dense connective tissue forms septa that separate lobules; adipose connective tissue is scant	Dense connective tissue capsule is present	Dense connective tissue is only found surrounding bronchioles and bronchi

	Vagina	Esophagus
Epithelia	Both nonkeratinized stratified squamous epithelium	
Lamina propria	No glands are present	Contain glands
Muscularis	Smooth muscles only	Skeletal muscles may be observed in the upper two-thirds of the esophagus

Special Sensory System | 15

INTRODUCTION

Vision, smell, taste, hearing, and sense of balance are detected and interpreted by a set of specialized sensory organs and receptors. The eyes are specialized to let in the light, refract it, and focus it onto the special sensory receptors on the retina. The ears are composed of three sets of structures designed to channel sound waves toward the sensory receptors found in the inner ear. The inner ear is also responsible for sensing and maintaining balance and interpreting linear and angular acceleration. Taste is detected by the taste buds in the oral cavity (covered in the Digestive System section). Olfactory receptors in the superior concha of the nasal cavity receive and transfer odoriferous information to the central nervous system (CNS; covered in the Respiratory System section).

THE SPECIAL SENSORY SYSTEM

EYE		
Structure	**Function**	**Location**
Macroscopic features		
Paired globular organ; three tunics	Collecting, channeling, refracting light to focus on the retina for visual stimuli	Orbital cavity in the skull
1. Fibrous tunic: Tough, dense, and thick layer	1. Forming a tough, rigid outer lining	1. Outermost layer of the eye
a. Cornea: Clear, highly convex region of the fibrous tunic	a. Refracting light into the globe	a. Anterior one-sixth of the fibrous tunic

(continued)

EYE (continued)

Structure		Function	Location

Macroscopic features

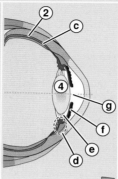

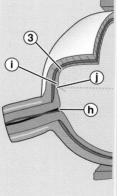

b. Sclera: Majority of the fibrous tunic; white and gray	b. Protecting, giving rigidity to the eye, serving as attachment site for extrinsic muscles of the eye	b. Rest of the five-sixths of the fibrous tunic
2. Vascular (uveal) tunic: Dark, thinner layer containing melanocytes and vasculature	2. Delivery of vascular supply to the inner eye	2. Deep to fibrous tunic, middle layer of the eye
c. Choroid: Majority of vascular tunic; thin, dark layer	c. Limiting scattering of light within the globe	c. Posterior four-sixths of the vascular tunic
d. Ciliary body: Thickened ring of vascular tunic that projects into the vitreous chamber	d. Participating in accommodation, producing aqueous humor	d. Ring of vascular tunic between iris and choroid, at the same plane as the lens
e. Suspensory ligaments: Series of thin fibers	e. Pulling or releasing the lens in the process of accommodation	e. Run between ciliary body and peripheral rim of the lens

Structure		Function	Location
Macroscopic features			
f. Iris: Anterior-most rim of the vascular tunic		f. Adjusting the diameter of the pupil	f. Anterior one-sixth of the vascular tunic, in front of the lens
g. Pupil: Opening in the center of the iris		g. Allowing the light to enter the globe	g. In the middle of the iris
3. Retina: Thin, translucent, yellowish layer		3. Sensing the light stimuli and transferring the information to the CNS	3. Innermost layer of the eye
h. Optic disc: Slightly depressed region of the retina where optic nerve exits the eye		h. Serving as an exit point for all axons	h. Slightly medial to fovea centralis
i. Fovea centralis: Slightly thinner region of the retina		i. Reception of visual information with high acuity	i. Medial to optic disc, in line with the pupil
j. Macula densa: Thinnest region of the retina		j. Reception of visual information with the highest acuity	j. Center of the fovea centralis
4. Lens: Oval, translucent structure		4. Fine refraction of light to focus it on macula densa	4. At the center of the ciliary body

(continued)

EYE (continued)		
Structure	Function	Location
Macroscopic features		
5. Anterior chamber: Space filled with aqueous humor	5. Containing aqueous humor	5. Between cornea and iris
6. Posterior chamber: Space filled with aqueous humor	6. Containing aqueous humor	6. Between iris and lens
7. Vitreous cavity: Space filled with gelatinous vitreous humor	7. Containing vitreous humor	7. Posterior to the lens

FIBROUS TUNIC		
Structure	Function	Location
Cornea		
1. Corneal (anterior) epithelium: Nonkeratinized stratified squamous, about five layers of cells with abundant free nerve endings	1. Protection of the cornea, eliciting blinking and tearing response to touch	1. Anterior-most layer of the cornea
2. Bowman membrane: Thick acellular modified basement membrane	2. Providing strength to cornea, preventing infection spread	2. Deep to corneal epithelium, only in cornea
3. Corneal stroma (substantia propria): Thickest, 90% of the cornea, parallel layers of collagen fibrils	3. Contributing to transparency of the cornea	3. Between the Bowman and Descemet membranes

Structure		Function	Location
Cornea			
4. Descemet membrane: Thick basement membrane of the endothelium		4. Supporting endothelium, separating it from the stroma	4. Between corneal stroma and endothelium
5. Endothelium: Simple squamous epithelium		5. Engaging in metabolic exchange between cornea and aqueous humor	5. Innermost layer in contact with aqueous humor of the anterior chamber
Corneoscleral limbus			
			Junction of cornea and sclera
6. Thickened anterior epithelium		6. Housing stem cells for corneal epithelium	6. Anteriormost layer
7. Abrupt disappearance of Bowman membrane		7. Blending of stromal tissue with scleral connective tissue	7. Deep to anterior epithelium
8. Trabecular meshwork: Irregular channels lined with endothelium		8. Draining and conducting aqueous humor toward canal of Schlemm	8. Stromal layer
9. Scleral venous sinus (canal of Schlemm): Large channel formed by convergence of trabecular meshwork		9. Larger drainage for aqueous humor	9. Throughout corneoscleral limbus

(continued)

FIBROUS TUNIC (continued)			
Structure		**Function**	**Location**
Sclera			
10. Thick leathery layer, dense irregular connective tissue: Fiber bundles run in various directions but in parallel plane to each other		10. Protection, contributing to maintenance of the ocular pressure, allowing muscular attachments	10. Posterior five-sixths of the fibrous tunic

Additional Concepts

- **Vitreous humor:** Produces enough internal pressure and bulk to maintain the shape of the eye while allowing light to pass through hence is an important part of the structure of the eye.
- **Aqueous humor:** Circulates through the anterior cavity of the eye, delivering oxygen and nutrients to avascular structures such as the lens and the cornea.

Clinical Significance

- **LASIK:** A procedure to correct myopia by performing a corrective surgery on the cornea. Surgeons make an incision at the limbus, through the corneal stroma, and precisely shave off angles or spots and then replace the flap over it.
- **Glaucoma:** Increased intraocular pressure most commonly as the result of insufficient drainage of aqueous humor by the canal of Schlemm; if allowed to progress, the increased pressure on the retina reduces blood supply to the retina, resulting in blindness.
- **Floaters:** Translucent, coiled fibers present in one's visual field for a varying amount of time. These are tangled or denatured fibrous proteins of the vitreous humor. A few floaters do not have clinical significance and increase with age.

MNEMONIC

The mnemonic **ABCDE** can help you remember the layers of the cornea from anterior to posterior.

- **A**nterior epithelium
- **B**owman membrane
- **C**orneal stroma
- **D**escemet membrane
- **E**ndothelium

VASCULAR TUNIC			
Structure		**Function**	**Location**
Iris			
A diaphragm anterior to the lens		Adjusting the amount of light entering the eye	Anterior-most rim, between anterior and posterior chambers of the eye
1. Stroma: Well-vascularized connective tissue		1. Delivering nutrients to the iris	1. Anterior surface of the iris
a. Melano-cytes: Dark brown cells		a. Absorbing light, imparting eye color	a. Scattered through-out stroma
2. Two layers of pigment epithe-lium: Dark layer of cells contain-ing melanin granules		2. Absorbing light, con-tributing to eye color	2. Posterior surface of the iris
3. Sphincter pupillae: Ring of smooth muscle cells		3. Contracting to decrease pupil size	3. Circle around the pupil within stromal layer
4. Dilator pupillae: Smooth mus-cles arranged radially		4. Contracting to increase pupil size	4. Peripheral to sphincter pupillae, anterior to pigment epithelium
5. Pupil: Central aperture		5. Opening through which light enters the eye	5. Center of iris
Ciliary body			
Thickened ring of vascular tunic		Aqueous humor produc-tion, participation in accom-modation	Between iris and choroid

(continued)

VASCULAR TUNIC (continued)

Structure		Function	Location
Ciliary body			
6. Ciliary processes: Radial ridges and projections into posterior chamber	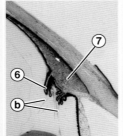	6. Anchoring zonular fibers, participation in aqueous humor production	6. Extending out into posterior chamber
b. Suspensory ligaments (zonular fibers): Thin, translucent fibers arising from ciliary processes		b. Attachment to the lens, participation in accommodation	b. Run between ciliary processes and peripheral rim of the lens
7. Ciliary muscles: Smooth muscles		7. Main participant in accommodation	7. Within ciliary body
Choroid			
Thin sheet of dark brown tissue	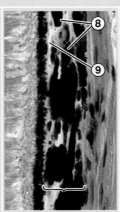	Delivery of nutrient and prevention of light reflection	Between sclera and retina
8. Melanocytes: Dark brown cells		8. Pigment production	8. Scattered throughout choroid
9. Bruch membrane: Thin, acellular layer		9. Forming a boundary between choroid and retina, firmly anchoring retina to choroid	9. Between choroid and retina

Additional Concepts

- **Parasympathetic innervation of the iris**
  - **Sphincter pupillae:** Innervated by the parasympathetic nerve; hence, in a relaxed state, parasympathetic signals contract sphincter pupillae, reducing the size of the pupil.
  - **Dilator pupillae:** Innervated by the sympathetic nerve; hence, under stressful conditions, sympathetic signals contract dilator pupillae and increase the size of the pupil.
- **Accommodation:** Ability to regulate convexity of lens to fine tune the refraction of light, ensuring image is focused on fovea centralis. Accommodation is achieved by the contraction of ciliary muscles.
  - Focusing on an up-close object: Ciliary muscles contract, making the diameter of the opening in the middle of the ciliary body smaller. Zonula fibers are relaxed and lens is allowed to be rounded due to its elastic nature. Sore eyes when staring at a nearby object are thought to be caused by lactic acid buildup in the ciliary muscles as the result of prolonged contraction.
  - Focusing on a far-away object: Ciliary muscles relax, increasing the diameter of the opening in the middle of the ciliary body. Zonular fibers become taught and pull on the periphery of the lens, and the lens flattens.

Clinical Significance

- **Uveal melanoma:** Melanoma that arises from the melanocytes of the uvea (vascular tunic). Though rare, uveal melanomas are highly malignant tumors that tend to metastasize most commonly to the liver via blood vessels. The size of the tumor and its breach of the Bruch membrane affect patients' prognosis.

RETINA			
Structure		Function	Location
Pigmented layer			
1. Retinal pigment epithelium: Simple cuboidal epithelium		1. Absorbing excess light to prevent reflection, photosensitivity restoration, phagocytosis of debris	Outer layer of retina, attached to Bruch membrane

(continued)

RETINA (continued)

Structure		Function	Location
Pigmented layer			
a. Abundant zonula occludens and gap junctions		a. Forming blood-retina barrier	
Neural layer (neural retina, retina proper)			
Nine layers formed by photoreceptor cells, interneurons, and glial cells		Receive and transmit visual sensory stimuli	Outermost layer
2. Photoreceptors (rods and cones)		2. Responding, initiating action potential in response to photons	
3. Exterior (outer) limiting membrane		3. Forming a boundary of supporting cells	
4. Outer nuclear layer: Cell bodies of rods and cones		4. Containing cell bodies of rods and cones	
5. Outer plexiform layer: Cell process of rods, cones, and other neurons		5. Housing processes of rods, cones, and other interneurons; allowing synapses	

Structure	Function	Location
Neural layer (neural retina, retina proper)		
6. Inner nuclear layer: Cell bodies of other neurons	6. Containing cell bodies of inter-neurons	
7. Inner plexi-form layer: Cell processes	7. Housing pro-cesses of inter-neurons, allow-ing synapses	
8. Ganglion cell layer: Cell bodies of ganglion cells	8. Containing cell bodies of gan-glion cells that conduct signals	
9. Nerve fiber layer: Thin ganglion cell processes	9. Containing ganglion cell pro-cesses, conduct-ing visual signals to the brain	
10. Inner limiting membrane: Basal lamina	10. Forming acellu-lar layer between retina and vitre-ous chamber	Innermost layer

Clinical Significance

- **Detached retina:** Loose connection between the two layers of the retina is a potential space between neural and pigmented layer of the retina. Treatment includes introduction of air bubbles and prone positioning of the head for a prolonged time to help push the neural layer against the pigmented layer until the contact is re-established.

MNEMONIC

In New Generation It Is Only Ophthalmologist Examines Patient's Retina: Retinal layers from inside to outside

In (Inner limiting membrane)
New (Nerve fiber layer)
Generation (Ganglion cell)
It (Inner plexiform layer)
Is (Inner nuclear layer)
Only (Outer plexiform layer)
Ophthalmologist (Outer nuclear layer)
Examines (Exterior limiting membrane)
Patient's (Photoreceptors, rods, cones)
Retina (Retinal pigment epithelium)

LENS

Structure	Function	Location
Macroscopic features		
Biconvex, transparent, avascular crystalline structure 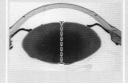	Refract the light and find tune the focus onto fovea centralis	Suspended by zonular fibers at the level of ciliary body, between posterior and vitreous chambers
Microscopic structures		
1. Lens capsule: Thick, modified basement membrane 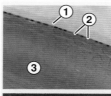	1. Forming the boundary, protecting the lens, providing attachment sites for zonular fibers	1. Surround the entire surface of the lens
2. Subcapsular epithelium: Simple cuboidal epithelium	2. Giving rise to new lens fibers	2. Only on the anterior surface, deep to lens capsule
3. Lens fibers: Thin, elongated, flattened structures filled with crystalline proteins and precisely aligned with each other • No simple epithelial lining on posterior surface	3. Imparting transparency and refractory property to lens	3. Form the bulk of the lens

Clinical Significance

- **Cataract:** Gradual, progressive loss of transparency of the lens associated with increasing age. Abnormalities in lens crystalline proteins and fiber organization have been observed in opaque lenses of cataract patients. Replacement of the effected lens with an artificial lens is indicated in advanced cases of cataract with significant vision impairment.
- **Presbyopia:** Far-sightedness that develops with loss of elasticity in the lens and the ability to accommodate, resulting in inability to focus on nearby objects.

EAR			
Structure		**Function**	**Location**
Macroscopic features			
1. External ear: Visible and easily accessible portions		1. Sound collection, localization, conduction to middle ear	1. Lateral sides of the head approximately at the level of the eyes
a. Auricle (pinna): Outward appendage of varying shape and size		a. Sound collection, localization	a. External protrusion
b. External auditory meatus: Air-filled channel, containing hair and modified sebaceous glands (ceruminous glands)		b. Sound wave conduction, trapping foreign particles	b. Internal tubule running toward middle ear

(continued)

EAR (continued)

Structure	Function	Location
Macroscopic features		

c. Tympanic membrane: Thin, transparent membrane

   c. Vibration and conversion of sound energy into mechanical energy

   c. Between external and middle ear

2. Middle ear: Air-filled space containing three ossicles

   2. Transmission of mechanical energy to inner ear

   2. Within the petrous portion of temporal bone

d. Malleus: Small bone in contact with tympanic membrane

   d. Transferring mechanical energy from tympanic membrane to malleus

   d. Between tympanic membrane and incus

e. Incus: Largest of three ossicles in the middle

   e. Transferring energy from malleus to stapes

   e. Between malleus and stapes

f. Stapes: Bone in contact with oval window

   f. Vibrating in and out on oval window of the inner ear

   f. Between incus and oval window

g. Auditory tube: Narrow, flattened tube that may be opened to equalize middle ear pressure

   g. Maintaining appropriate air pressure within the middle ear

   g. Between middle ear and nasopharynx

Structure		Function	Location
Macroscopic features			
3. Inner ear: Structure of complex shape		3. Containing special sensory receptors for hearing and balance	3. Within petrous portion of temporal bone, medial to middle ear
h. Semicircular canals: Three bony arches		h. Housing semicircular canals	h. Posterior to middle ear
i. Vestibule: Oval, mid-structure		i. Housing utricle and saccule	i. Antero-medial to semicircular canals
j. Cochlea: Spiral-shaped bony casing		j. Housing cochlear duct	j. Medial to middle ear
4. Vestibulo-cochlear nerve		4. Conducting special sensory information to CNS	4. Runs between cochlea and the brain

Clinical Significance

- **Middle ear infection:** Auditory tube is normally collapsed and approximately 3.5 cm in length in adults. It is, however, significantly shorter in infants, making them susceptible to spread of infection from the pharynx to the middle ear through the auditory tube, which results in otitis media.
- **Conducting hearing loss:** Results from the mechanical failure in transmitting sound to the otherwise normal inner ear. The problem thus may involve any structures in the external and middle ears including otitis media, excess earwax, and otosclerosis. Conducting hearing loss may be treatable by medical or surgical interventions.
- **Sensorineural hearing loss/impairment:** Results from damage to or dysfunctional sensory receptors, the cochlear nerve, or the auditory nerve pathway. Sensorineuronal impairment accounts for about 90% of hearing. Cochlear implants may restore some auditory function in select patients.

INNER EAR		
Structure	Function	Location
Bony labyrinth		
Outer, bony casing of the inner ear, containing membranous labyrinth suspended in perilymph	Housing, protecting, insulating membranous labyrinth	Outer layer of the inner ear
1. Semicircular canals: Three arches in three different planes	1. Housing semicircular ducts	1. Posterior to middle ear
2. Vestibule: Oval swelling	2. Housing utricle and saccule	2. Antero-medial to semicircular canals
3. Cochlea: Snail shell–like spiral structure	3. Housing cochlear duct	3. Medial to middle ear
Membranous labyrinth		
Thin, delicate, translucent series of tubule systems suspended in the perilymph of bony labyrinth. Filled with endolymph, containing special sensory structures	Housing endolymph and special sensory structures for hearing and sense of balance	Suspended within the perilymph of the bony labyrinth
4. Semicircular ducts: Three arches	4. Detection of angular movements	4. Within semicircular canal
a. Cristae ampullaris: Thickened epithelial ridge containing hair cells	a. Housing sensory hair cells	a. At each base of semicircular ducts

Structure		Function	Location
Membranous labyrinth			
b. Copula: Gelatinous mass		b. Bending hair cells embedded in it to trigger action potential	b. A thickened spot on the wall of each ampulla
5. Utricle: Dilated, oval structure		5. Detection of linear movements	5. Within vestibule, closer to semicircular duct
c. Macula: Thickened epithelial ridge		c. Housing sensory hair cells	c. A thickened spot on utricular wall
d. Otolith membrane: Gelatinous mass with crystalline particles (otoliths)		d. Bending hair cells embedded in it to trigger action potential	d. On top of and in contact with macula
6. Saccule: Dilated oval structure with macula and otolith membrane		6. Detection of vertical movements	6. Within vestibule, closer to cochlear duct
7. Cochlear duct (scala media): Thin tube coiled 2.5 turns		7. Detection of sound	7. Within cochlea
e. Vestibular membrane: Two simple squamous epithelia with basement membrane in between		e. Forming the roof of cochlear duct	e. Top layer of cochlear duct

(continued)

INNER EAR (continued)		
Structure	Function	Location
Membranous labyrinth		
f. Basilar membrane: Contains organ of Corti on top of basement membrane and simple squamous epithelium	f. Forming the base of cochlear duct, housing organ of Corti	f. Bottom layer of cochlear duct
g. Organ of Corti: Two rows of hair cells and supporting cells	g. Housing sensory hair cells	g. On basilar membrane, throughout the length of cochlear duct
h. Tectorial membrane: Sheet of collagen fibers	h. Bending of hair cells embedded in it to trigger action potential	h. Within cochlear duct, in contact with hair cells of organ of Corti

8. Scala vestibule: Perilymph-filled space above vestibular membrane	8. Transmitting energy from oval window to helicotrema	8. Space between cochlear wall and vestibular membrane
9. Helicotrema: Connecting point between scala vestibuli and tympani, filled with perilymph	9. Connecting perilymph-filled spaces between scala vestibuli and tympani, allowing energy transmission	9. At the tip of cochlear spiral

Structure	Function	Location
Membranous labyrinth		
10. Scala tympani: Perilymph-filled space below basilar membrane	10. Transmitting energy from helicotrema to round window, vibrating basilar membrane	10. Space between cochlear wall and basilar membrane

All sources are published by Lippincott Williams & Wilkins unless otherwise noted.

CHAPTER 1

Page 2, top to bottom Cui D. *Atlas of Histology with Functional and Clinical Correlations,* 2011, Fig. 2-8B, p. 21; Eroschenko VP. *diFiore's Atlas of Histology with Functional Correlations,* 12th ed., 2013, Fig. 1.2, p. 4; Eroschenko, Fig. 1.2, p. 4; Courtesy of Lisa M. J. Lee, PhD, Department of Cell and Developmental Biology, University of Colorado School of Medicine.
Page 3 Ross MH, Pawlina W. *Histology: A Text and Atlas,* 6th ed., 2011, Fig. 2.45, p. 60.
Page 4, top to bottom Cui, Fig. 2-8A, p. 21; Cui, Fig. 3-1A, p. 19; Eroschenko, Fig. 2.6, p. 25.
Page 5, top to bottom Eroschenko, Fig. 2.10, p. 29; Eroschenko, Fig. 2.7, p. 27.
Page 6, top to bottom Cui, Fig. 3-1A, p. 19; Cui, Fig. 2-2, p. 15; Ross, Fig. 2.46, p. 61; Ross MH, Pawlina W. *Histology: A Text and Atlas,* 6th ed., 2011, Fig. 2.49, p. 63.
Page 7, top to bottom Ross MH, Pawlina W. *Histology: A Text and Atlas,* 6th ed., 2011, Fig. 2.40, p. 58; Ross, Fig. 2.55, p. 70; Ross, Fig. 2.52, p. 69.
Page 8, top to bottom Cui, Fig. 2-8B, p. 21; Ross, Fig. 2.45, p. 60; Ross, Fig. 1.4, p. 8.
Page 9, top to bottom Gartner LP, Hiatt JL. *Color Atlas of Histology,* 5th ed. 2009, Fig. 2, p. 45; Gartner, Fig. 1, p. 21.

CHAPTER 2

Page 12, top to bottom Cui, Fig. 2-6A, p. 19; Ross, Fig. 5.22, p. 133.
Page 13, top to bottom Ross, Fig. 5.28, p. 138; Cui, Fig. 3-1A, p. 29.
Page 14 Cui, Fig. 3-1A, p. 29.
Page 15, top to bottom Cui, Fig. 3-1A, p. 29; Cui, Fig. 3-11B, p. 39; Cui, Fig. 3-11A, p. 39; Cui, Fig. 3-11C.
Page 16 Cui, Fig. 3-1A, p. 29.

CHAPTER 3

CHAPTER 4

CHAPTER 5

CHAPTER 6

Page 86, top to bottom Cui, Fig. 8-7B, p. 143; Cui, Fig. 8.2A, p. 138.
Page 87 Ross, Fig. 10.3, p. 272.
Page 88 Cui, Fig. 9-2, p. 159.
Page 89 Ross, Fig. 13.4, p. 402.
Page 90, top to bottom Gartner, Fig. 1, p. 175; Cui, Fig. 9-3C, p. 160.
Page 91 Gartner, Graphic 8-1, p. 162.
Page 92, top to bottom Gartner, Graphic 8-1, p. 162; Cui, Fig. 9-7B, p. 164.
Page 93, top to bottom Gartner, Fig. 1, p. 169; Cui, Fig. 9-8C, p. 164.
Page 94, top to bottom Cui, Fig. 9-10B, p. 167; Gartner, Fig. 2, p. 173.
Page 95, top to bottom Eroschenko, Fig. 10.3, p. 223; Cui, Fig. 9-13B, p. 170; Eroschenko, Fig. 10.4, p. 223.
Page 96, top to bottom Cui, Fig. 9-14B, p. 171; Cui, Fig. 9-14B, p. 171.
Page 97, top to bottom Gartner, Fig. 2, p. 173; Cui, Fig. 9-17C, p. 174.
Page 98 Cui, Fig. 9-17C, p. 174.

CHAPTER 7

Page 101 Gartner, Fig. 3, p. 311.
Page 102 Gartner, Fig. 4, p. 195.
Page 103, top to bottom Ross, Fig. 14.15a, p. 460; Ross, Fig. 14.15b, p. 460.
Page 104 Cui, Fig. 10-8A, p. 189.
Page 105 Eroschenko, Fig. 13.7, p. 293.
Page 106, top to bottom Cui, Fig. 10.10, p. 191; Cui, Fig. 10.11A, p. 192.
Page 107 Cui, Fig. 10.11B, p. 192.
Page 108 Cui, Fig. 10.10, p. 191.
Page 109, top to bottom Gartner, Fig. 1, p. 199; Cui, Fig. 10-13B, p. 194.
Page 110 Cui, Fig. 10-13C, p. 194.
Page 111 Cui, Fig. 10-14A, p. 195.
Page 112, top to bottom Gartner, Fig. 2, p. 201; Cui, Fig. 10-14C, p. 195.

CHAPTER 8

Pages 115 and 116 Cui, Fig. 13-3B, p. 246.
Page 117 Gartner, Fig. 3, p. 239.
Page 118 Gartner, Fig. 2, p. 239.
Page 119, top to bottom Ross, Fig. 15.12, p. 503; Gartner, Fig. 3, p. 243.

CHAPTER 9

CHAPTER 10

CHAPTER 11

Page 179, top to bottom Gartner, Fig. 4, p. 344; Eroschenko, Fig. 18.11, p. 439.
Pages 180 and 181 Cui, Fig. 12-8B, p. 231.
Page 182 Eroschenko, Fig. 18.7, p. 435.
Pages 183 and 184 Ross, Fig. 20.24, p. 723.
Page 185 Eroschenko, Fig. 18.14, p. 441.
Page 186 Gartner, Fig. 2, p. 351.
Page 187, top to bottom Cui, Fig. 12.1, p. 224; Gartner, Fig. 3, p. 351; Gartner, Fig. 4, p. 351.

CHAPTER 12

Page 189 Gartner, Fig. 1, p. 215.
Page 190 Gartner, Fig. 1, p. 215; Cui, Fig. 17.4B, p. 330.
Page 191 Gartner, Fig. 1, p. 215.
Page 192 Cui, Fig. 17.6B, p. 332.
Page 193 Cui, Fig. 17-5B, p. 331.
Page 194 Cui, Fig. 17.10A, p. 336.
Page 195 Cui, Fig. 17.10B, p. 336.
Page 196, top to bottom Gartner, Plate 10-3, p. 218; Cui, Fig. 17-8A, p. 334.
Page 197 Cui, Fig. 17-8B, p. 334.
Page 198, top to bottom Cui, Fig. 17.9A, p. 335; Cui, Fig. 17.9B, p. 335.
Page 199, top to bottom Cui, Fig. 17.13A, p. 339; Cui, Fig. 17.13B, p. 339.

CHAPTER 13

Page 201 Ross, Fig. 22.4a, p. 790.
Page 202, top to bottom Cui, Fig. 18-14A, p. 360; Cui, Fig. 18-13A, p. 359.
Page 203, top to bottom Gartner, Fig. 4, p. 387; Cui, Fig. 18-7B, p. 353.
Page 204, top to bottom Gartner, Fig. 4, p. 387; Cui, Fig. 18-7B, p. 353; Gartner, Fig. 2, p. 389.
Page 205, top to bottom Ross, Fig. 22.6, p. 791; Ross, Fig. 22.4a, p. 790.
Page 206, top to bottom Eroschenko, Fig. 20.9, p. 489; Gartner, Fig. 4, p. 389.
Page 207 Cui, Fig. 18-19A, p. 365.
Page 208, top to bottom Gartner, Plate 18-4, p. 392; Gartner, Fig. 3, p. 391; Cui, Fig. 7-22A, p. 128.

Page 209 Cui, Fig. 18-20A, p. 366.
Page 210, top to bottom Gartner, Plate 18-4, p. 392; Cui, Fig. 18-22, p. 368.
Page 211 Gartner, Fig. 4, p. 393.

CHAPTER 14

Page 213 Cui, Fig. 19-3A, p. 374.
Page 214 Cui, Fig. 19.3A, p. 374.
Page 215, top to bottom Gartner, Fig. 3, p. 361; Gartner, Fig. 4, p. 361; Cui, Fig. 19-6B, p. 377.
Page 216, top to bottom Cui, Fig. 19-6B, p. 377; Gartner, Fig. 3, p. 361.
Page 217, top to bottom Gartner, Fig. 3, p. 361; Gartner, Fig. 4, p. 361; Cui, Fig. 19-6B, p. 377.
Page 218, top to bottom Cui, Fig. 19-7A, p. 378; Cui, Fig. 19-7B, p. 378.
Page 220 Gartner, Graphic 17-1, p. 354.
Page 221 Gartner, Fig. 1, p. 369.
Page 222, top to bottom Gartner, Fig. 2, p. 369; Gartner, Fig. 1, p. 371.
Page 223, top to bottom Gartner, Fig. 1, p. 369; Cui, Fig. 19-10B, p. 381.
Page 224, top to bottom Eroschenko, Fig. 21.16, p. 529; Cui, Fig. 19-10C, p. 381; Cui, Fig. 19-10A, p. 381.
Page 225, top to bottom Cui, Fig. 19-12A, p. 383; Ross, Fig. 23.21, p. 855.
Page 226, top to bottom Ross, Fig. 23.21, p. 855; Gartner, Graphic 17-1, p. 354.
Page 227, top to bottom Cui, Fig. 19-9A, p. 380; Gartner, Fig. 2, p. 367.
Page 228, top to bottom Cui, Fig. 19-14B, p. 385; Gartner, Fig. 4, p. 373.
Page 229 Cui, Fig. 19-15A, p. 386.
Page 230, top to bottom Eroschenko, Fig. 21.29, p. 551; Cui, Fig. 19-15B, p. 386.
Page 231, top to bottom Cui, Fig. 19-15C, p. 386; Eroschenko, Fig. 21.32, p. 555.

CHAPTER 15

Pages 235 and 236 Cui, Fig. 20-1, p. 392.
Page 237 Cui, Fig. 20-7A, p. 398.
Page 238, top to bottom Cui, Fig. 20-7A, p. 398, Cui, Fig. 20-5A, p. 396.

Page 239, top to bottom Cui, Fig. 20-5A, p. 396; Ross, Plate 107, p. 927.
Page 240 Eroschenko, Fig. 22.8, p. 569.
Page 241 Cui, Fig. 20-9B, p. 400.
Page 242, top to bottom Cui, Fig. 14-6A, p. 264; Gartner, Fig. 2, p. 407.
Page 244 Gartner, Fig. 2, p. 407.
Page 246, top to bottom Cui, Fig. 20-7A, p. 398; Cui, Fig. 20-7B, p. 398; Cui, Fig. 20-7C, p. 398.
Page 247 Cui, Fig. 21-1A, p. 412.
Page 248, top to bottom Cui, Fig. 21-1A, p. 412; Cui, Fig. 21-1B, p. 412.
Page 249 Cui, Fig. 21-1A, p. 412.
Page 250, top to bottom Cui, Fig. 21-2, p. 413; Cui, Fig. 21-8B, p. 419.
Page 251 Cui, Fig. 21-5, p. 416.
Page 252 Cui, Fig. 21-5, p. 416.

Note: Page numbers followed by "f" denote figures.